Living with

Klinefelter Syndrome (47,XXY)
Trisomy X (47,XXX)
and 47,XYY

Living with

Klinefelter Syndrome (47,XXY) Trisomy X (47,XXX) and 47,XYY

A guide for families and individuals affected by X and Y chromosome variations

Virginia Isaacs Cover MSW

New York

Published by:
Virginia Isaacs Cover
www.KlinefelterTrisomyX47XYY.com

Diagrams Meiosis and Mitosis by Patti Isaacs, www.parrotgraphics.com
Karyotypes provided by Wisconsin State Laboratory of Hygiene, Board of Regents of the University of Wisconsin Systems and Colorado Genetics
Cover image of DNA helix from iStockphoto.com
Book design by Dorie McClelland, www.springbookdesign.com

Printed in Canada by Friesens.

ISBN: 978-0-615-57400-4

I dedicate this book to the memory of my parents,
George Isaacs and Florence Higgins Isaacs

Contents

Introduction

Our journey with Klinefelter syndrome began in the spring of 1987. I was 38 and four months pregnant with a very much wanted second child, after a number of years of trying to conceive. We had followed the standard recommendation to have amniocentesis because of my "advanced maternal age." Several weeks later, I received a phone call at work from my obstetrician. She told me that the amniocentesis had shown that I was carrying a boy, and that he had an extra X chromosome, a condition called Klinefelter syndrome.

I remember that conversation now as if it had occurred this morning. It is one of the events in my life seared into my memory, much like learning in seventh grade that President Kennedy had been shot, or hearing in the coffee room at work that an airliner had flown into one of the twin towers of the World Trade Center. I remember asking my obstetrician if I could put her on hold to take the call in my office, closing the door, and picking up the phone again at my desk. The doctor asked me if I knew anything about this condition. I told her that I remembered the genetic counselor telling us what the amniocentesis would be looking for, including Down syndrome and other more severe trisomy conditions, which is the presence of three chromosomes where there should be only a pair of two. I had remembered the counselor telling us that sometimes they see extra sex chromosomes, but I had never given it another thought after the procedure. This seemed to be the case with my son, and I sat there trying to absorb it.

This physician had been my gynecologist for five years, and had seen me through a number of years of infertility testing and treatment. She had been overjoyed with us when we inexplicably achieved a pregnancy on our own. Now she was telling me that Klinefelter syndrome can cause a wide range of functioning, from barely impaired to more severely affected. It was associated with somewhat lower IQ compared to siblings. Klinefelter men could be tall, but not always. They often had speech delay and learning disabilities, and sometimes behavioral problems and difficulties with fine and gross motor skills. And they were always infertile.

She told me that she had already arranged for my husband and me to meet with the medical geneticist, along with our genetic counselor that afternoon. My obstetrician also told me that abortion was an option, but since I was already at eighteen weeks, she would want to do this immediately if this is what we chose. Then she told me that, although he did not have this genetic disorder, her oldest son had a similar range of disabilities, and if we wanted to discuss raising a child with mild or moderate deficits, she would be happy to talk with us.

That afternoon, we met with the geneticist, who explained Klinefelter syndrome, showing us the photo of the chromosomes, called a karyotype, while we both cried. She and the genetic counselor had photocopied a number of articles and chapters of books that described the results of longitudinal studies of groups of children with sex chromosome aneuploidy, and they talked with us about the studies and what they could tell us about how our baby might be affected. I did not know at the time that this sort of compassionate and knowledgeable counseling was so rare. They were telling us that with Klinefelter syndrome there are often developmental and learning challenges but that when families are prepared to support their children with speech therapy, additional help with schoolwork, adapted sports programs, and a warm and nurturing family life, a child with this condition can be expected to do well. For families like ours (my husband, Al, is a political science professor and I hold masters degrees in both social work and business administration), the counselor suggested that we might have to adjust our expectations regarding careers, however, because our child might not want to or be able to get a college degree.

We left the meeting, however, quite certain that we wanted to continue the pregnancy. It did not matter to us whether our son became a Supreme Court justice, electrician, or truck driver; we just wanted a healthy and happy child, who felt good about himself. We went home and pored over the medical journal articles that we had been given. The range of functioning in the various longitudinal studies from Edinburgh, Toronto, and Yale was very broad, with IQs ranging from 50 to over 120, and descriptions of very well-adjusted children as well as those who had significant behavioral problems. But overall, the picture was of children in intact homes with good schooling who did quite well. We thought that we could probably provide the services that our child would need.

I now know, from speaking with hundreds of parents who also received a prenatal diagnosis, that our experience was unusual. Parents have told me numerous times of being informed that the child would probably be retarded, or would likely end up in prison. Other parents have been told that their fetus is a "monster" and that abortion is the only option. I sometimes hear that the genetic counselor was well-informed about Klinefelter syndrome and that the obstetrician was supportive of the parent's decision to continue the pregnancy, but more often parents are left to surf the Web looking for accurate and current information. Our diagnosis was pre-Internet, and yet the information available to laypersons continues to be limited and sketchy. It is just as possible to find questionable information predicting pedophilia and sexual deviancy today as it is to find more current and credible information based on the latest research.

Our son, Jonathan, was born December of 1987. He was a beautiful and sweet baby boy, certainly on the quiet side, and far less active than his older brother had been. By the age of twelve months, we could tell that he was not meeting his developmental milestones, and by fifteen months, he was enrolled in an intensive early intervention program. John then began making steady progress, putting together sentences by age three, and learning his letters, colors and numbers by four. He continued into a self-contained kindergarten, and was mainstreamed two years later into first grade. I will comment throughout this text on his development from childhood through adolescence and into early adulthood.

Although I continued to look for and find occasional articles updating my knowledge about Klinefelter syndrome, I really wanted to meet other families with a boy like ours. Because John had a fairly extensive schedule of therapy services, we had elected to tell our families about his extra X chromosome. My mother was the one who saw Melissa Aylstock's letter to Dear Abby regarding her son's diagnosis of Klinefelter syndrome, which was written in 1989. The national response to this letter inspired Melissa to found an organization, Klinefelters Syndrome and Associates (now KS&A), that began providing education and support for families and individuals affected by 47,XXY. In 1995, I attended a national conference in Chevy Chase, Maryland. It was the first time that I had ever met another family with a child with Klinefelter syndrome.

Over the next fifteen years, the national advocacy groups, KS&A and AAKSIS (American Association for Klinefelter Syndrome Information and Support), provided our most important source of information regarding Klinefelter syndrome and how to manage and treat the various educational and psychosocial issues associated with it. Klinefelter Syndrome &Associates, or KS&A, has since changed its name to stand for "Knowledge, Action and Support" and has broadened its approach to providing information and support to the other sex chromosome aneuploid conditions, 47,XYY, and 47,XXX, and their variations.

John had considerable educational challenges and developed a severe psychiatric disorder during adolescence. Other parents were the ones who helped us through these episodes. We learned from national conferences to consult the few medical specialists who had taken an interest in Klinefelter syndrome, and who were beginning to conduct research into the disorder.

I also became active in these organizations, and helped to organize and run the New York City area support group for ten years. And I was continually frustrated by the lack of awareness about Klinefelter syndrome in both the general population as well as among health care professionals. At some point, I thought, surely someone will publish a book, and update the information that Robert Bock of the National Institutes of Health wrote into his excellent brochure, "Understanding Klinefelter Syndrome," published in 1993.

Unfortunately, Klinefelter syndrome and the other SCA conditions of Trisomy X and XYY syndrome have never received the broad national attention and funding that other genetic disorders, such as autism and Down syndrome have. It did not appear that anyone else was prepared to undertake the work to write and publish a guide for families and individuals affected by these conditions.

I had developed writing skills through a long career as a social worker and health care administrator, working in the area of developmental disabilities. Having retired in September of 2010, I also had the time to devote to a guide written to be understandable by laypersons. This is my contribution to the sex chromosome aneuploidy ("SCA" is used throughout this guide as shorthand) community and to all the affected adults and children, to their families, friends and significant others, and to the professionals who chose to include specialization in Klinefelter syndrome and other SCA conditions in their practices and research.

This guide uses interviews that I conducted with family members of persons who have SCA as well as adults who have one of the SCA conditions. I also use quite a bit of information from a survey that I posted online from October 2010, through March 2011, on www.SurveyMonkey.com. This survey was publicized through e-mail and on websites to the membership of a number of SCA support groups. More than 800 individuals and families responded.

This was not a scientific survey but rather one focused on opinions, experience and educational needs. The results of the survey are referred to throughout the text. Quotations from answers provided by respondents illustrate the text and make the information more applicable to individual experiences. The findings from the survey will be summarized in a "webinar" that will be presented in early 2012 and thereafter will be available on the KS&A website, www.genetic.org.

The guide is not a research article, but rather provides information for affected individuals, their family members, and the professionals who work with them. It emphasizes the range of functioning and of symptoms that characterize the SCA conditions of 47,XXY; 47,XYY; 47,XXX, and variations of these disorders. I do provide the bibliography of scientific articles that I used to summarize functioning and best practices, but the text is not footnoted in the way that a peer-reviewed article would be.

While previous brief summaries have shied away from discussing the more controversial areas, such as overlap with autism spectrum disorders and concern that some XXY adults express about gender identity and sexual preference, this guide discusses what people have told me. It is not a scientific paper. My goal is to provide readable and accurate information, and to help families see their loved ones in the context of what others have experienced.

I use some shorthand in the guide. Sex chromosome aneuploidy is referred to as SCA. Klinefelter syndrome is shortened to KS. There are also other acronyms: EI (Early Intervention); IEP (Individualized Educational Plan); and ADHD (attention deficit hyperactivity disorder). Girls and women with 47,XXX, are often referred to as having Trisomy X.

Throughout this guide, Klinefelter syndrome is referred to as KS, or by its genetic signature, 47,XXY, or when appropriate, one of the variations, such as 48,XXXY. There is currently a fair amount of debate in the Klinefelter syndrome community about whether having the sex chromosome aneuploidy of 47,XXY, also means that the individual has Klinefelter syndrome. Syndrome refers to a collection of symptoms, and a person diagnosed with a syndrome may have one or many of the symptoms identified with a particular syndrome. The more symptoms, and the more pronounced particular symptoms are, the more severe the presentation of the syndrome.

The trisomy aneuploid conditions, 47,XXY, 47,XXX, and 47,XYY, are characterized by an enormous amount of variability in presentation. Many adults with these conditions are characteristically tall, but there is also a significant number who are of average or short stature. Similarly, although learning disabilities significant enough to require special education services affect about two-thirds, another third progress satisfactorily through school without any special assistance.

Several symptoms of Klinefelter syndrome, (47,XXY), are almost universal, however, including hypogonadism caused by testicular failure in early adulthood, and infertility. A tiny percentage of men with KS, probably not more than one or two percent, will escape even testicular failure and infertility or greatly lowered fertility. For this reason, there are many parents as well as adults who contend that having a genetic signature of 47,XXY, does not necessarily mean that a male has Klinefelter syndrome. In developing this guide, however, I will usually refer to this particular condition as KS, because I am assuming that the unaffected individual or his parents will not be interested in reading in detail about a syndrome from which he does not really suffer.

This guide also covers information regarding the variations of Klinefelter syndrome, including 48,XXXY; 48,XXYY; and 49,XXXXY. These variations tend to have a more severe presentation. Many parents believe that that the features of variations of KS are much more significant than in 47,XXY, and that they should be recognized as independent syndromes. There are many important similarities, however. They are rare and there has not been nearly the research on the variations as there has been on 47,XXY. The guide will provide summaries of what is available as well as information provided by families of these individuals.

In addition, I provide as much information as possible on 47,XYY, in males, and on 47,XXX, known as Trisomy X, in females, as well as the variations of SCA in females, 48,XXXX, and 49,XXXXX. Trisomy X and XYY conditions are somewhat less common that KS, and even less likely to be diagnosed properly. There also is considerably less research into these conditions. XYY and Trisomy X may not include the same level of endocrine disorder, infertility, or medical complications as KS. But there is considerable overlap in developmental and psychosocial issues including psychiatric co-morbidity, learning disability, and speech delay. Although initially, I had planned a guide covering Klinefelter syndrome only, I decided that failing to present what we do know about the other SCA conditions would be a lost opportunity to provide valuable information for these individuals and their families.

The content is meant to apply to all age groups, but the sad truth is that most articles about managing the features of SCA have been written about children and young adults. There is not a great deal of material that targets men and women with SCA much past early adulthood. The audience for much of the material is the parent, although I try to switch the voice when discussing adult issues, such as parenthood, sexual health, and work experience to speak to adults who are now independent. I hope that in the future I can write an updated edition that provides more guidance for those thirty and older, as well as addressing issues of middle and old age.

Virginia Isaacs Cover
December, 2011

What is Sex Chromosome Aneuploidy?

The most common abnormal chromosomal condition in humans is *sex chromosome aneuploidy* (SCA), or a variation in the usual number of sex chromosomes. Usually, there are 22 pairs of numbered chromosomes (from 1 to 22) and a pair of sex chromosomes (X or Y chromosomes) that normally give humans a total of 46 chromosomes. The usual sex chromosomes are one X and one Y in a male, or two X chromosomes in a female. In human males, the X and the Y chromosomes form a pair, with the mother's egg always contributing an X chromosome. The sex of the baby is determined by the sex chromosome of the father's sperm, which can contain either an X or a Y chromosome. If the father's sperm contributes a Y to the pair, the embryo develops as a male; if the sperm contributes an X to the pair, the embryo develops as a female.

When one extra chromosome is present, that pair is instead a threesome, known as a trisomy. Trisomies are often not survivable, and the embryo will spontaneously abort, or will be lost in miscarriage. Even when the trisomy condition is survivable, as it is with Trisomy 21 (Down syndrome) and Trisomy 18 (Edwards syndrome), the babies that are born have significant intellectual disability as well as serious health problems. SCA is the most survivable of the trisomies, and is not often associated with devastating disability. SCA affects an estimated 1 in 500 live births. By comparison, Down syndrome affects approximately 1 in 800 and Edwards Syndrome, only 1 in 6000.

Klinefelter syndrome (47,XXY), involving an additional X chromosome in a male, is the most common of these SCA conditions and is estimated to occur in approximately 1 in 600 male births. Less common SCA conditions include Trisomy X, (47,XXX) or a female with three X chromosomes, which occurs in approximately 1 in 1,000 female births, and 47,XYY, a male with two Y chromosomes, which occurs in approximately 1 in 1,000 male births. Other sex chromosome aneuploid conditions include variations of Klinefelter syndrome and Trisomy X where there are two or more additional X or Y chromosomes, instead of just one additional X or Y chromosome, and these are much less common.

In the most common form of Klinefelter syndrome, there are 47 chromosomes, with an additional X being the supernumerary chromosome. For that reason, it is given a genetic signature of 47,XXY, for the total number of chromosomes (47), and the trisomy of XXY, rather than the typical pair for a male of an X chromosome and a Y chromosome, which is given the genetic signature of 46,XY. Many individuals and professionals prefer to refer to Klinefelter syndrome as 47,XXY, but there are also many who use the term KS to refer to this condition. KS is used throughout this guide.

In Trisomy X, the genetic signature is 47,XXX. XYY has occasionally been called "Jacobs syndrome," but the condition is most commonly referred to as XYY syndrome, or just "XYY." It has a genetic signature of 47,XYY.

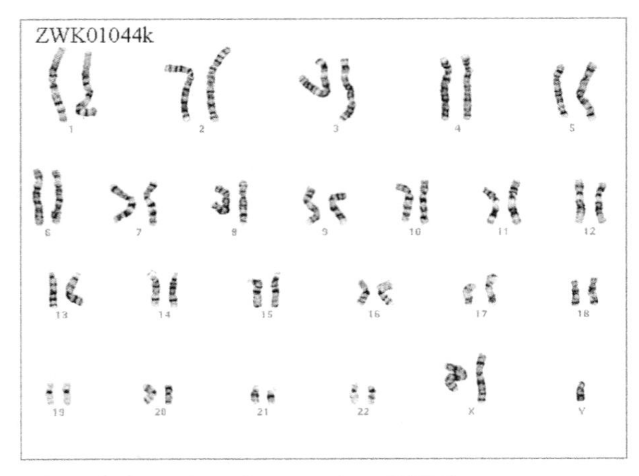

Klinefelter Syndrome (47,XXY)
Used with permission of the Wisconsin State Laboratory of Hygiene, Board of Regents of the University of Wisconsin System.

The most striking aspect of SCA is its variability in presentation, which is true for all of the trisomy conditions, XXY, XXX and XYY. The physical signs of SCA in babies and young children, if they are present, are often subtle and frequently overlooked by pediatricians, especially during "well-baby" checks, when attention must be paid to immunizations, vital signs, growth charts, and general development. Babies with other genetic syndromes are often dysmorphic, meaning that their facial features are unusual and that they have noticeable abnormalities in head shape and size, or an unusual appearance to eyes, ears, and nose, or extremities. But babies and children with SCA are not usually dysmorphic or unusual in their appearance; instead, they are often described as adorable. They are also frequently described as "easy" babies, sometimes quieter and less active than their siblings. One can imagine that this certainly makes them popular with parents!

When these individuals do have physical signs in early childhood, they are most often subtle, and include hypotonia, or low muscle tone, and as well as delays, often mild, in meeting developmental milestones, such as sitting, walking or talking. There can be learning disabilities in school, although nearly a third of those diagnosed in childhood have no special educational difficulties. Many are shy and withdrawn, or suffer from anxiety, ADHD or other emotional problems, but a significant number never have these challenges. Others progress unremarkably through their teens but have trouble holding jobs as adults. The majority experience success and happiness as adults, but admit that they were late bloomers who finished their education and became established in careers four to six years later than their peers.

Think of these disorders as "spectrum disorders" because there are some who have barely any physical signs, or educational challenges; there are many (the majority) who have some of the symptoms, but not all, and have mild/moderate presentations of the syndrome; and there is another minority that has a number of symptoms, some of which are severe and have a significant impact on their lives.

Both KS and Trisomy X also have variant forms in which there are 48 or 49 chromosomes. The variant forms tend to have more consistently severe symptoms. The genetic signatures for the variations of KS are 48,XXXY; 48,XXYY; and 49,XXXXY. The genetic signature for Tetrasomy X is 48,XXXX, and for Pentasomy X, 49,XXXXX. 47,XYY almost never occurs in a variant form, although there have been a few case reports of 48,XYYY, and 49,XXYYY.

There can also be mosaic forms of all of the conditions, meaning that the individual has two or more cell lines. A certain percentage of cells will have one number of X or Y chromosomes, while the remaining cells have a different number of X or Y chromosomes and thus a different total number of chromosomes in each of the "cell lines." This is called mosaicism because the different cell lines exist and fit together in the body like mosaic tiles in a piece of artwork. Most commonly, the individual has the typical number of X or Y chromosomes, 2, for a total of 46 chromosomes in one cell line. The other cell line has 3 sex chromosomes, and a total of 47 chromosomes in the second cell line. The genetic signature is then written (for Klinefelter syndrome) as 46,XY/47,XXY, or (for XYY syndrome) as 46,XY/47,XYY. Mosaicism can even involve the 48 and 49 chromosome variations, as in (for Trisomy X) 46,XX/47,XXX/48,XXXX.

In Trisomy X, it is not unusual that a mosaic presentation is 47,XXX/45,X. 45,X is also an aneuploid condition, but it is a monosomy, rather than a trisomy, and results in a condition called Turner syndrome. Turner syndrome, which can produce extremely complex medical problems, is not covered in this guide in any detail because its presentation is markedly different from the trisomy sex chromosome aneuploid conditions.

Turner syndrome, or 45,X, results when a female develops with only one X chromosome, instead of two X chromosomes. Girls and women with Turner syndrome usually have short stature, may have cardiac complications, and often have short, thickened and sometimes webbed necks. All women with Turner syndrome are sterile, although those with mosaic Turner syndrome may be able to become pregnant and bear children. It is estimated that only 1 in 100 Turner syndrome pregnancies results in a live birth. The rate of fetal demise is extraordinarily high, in contrast to the survivability of other sex chromosome aneuploid conditions that are discussed in this guide. Infants with Turner syndrome are usually identified shortly after birth because of their easily recognized physical characteristics. They often have cardiac problems, and they may also have distinct cognitive difficulties, which tend to be quite different from those of individuals with extra X and Y chromosomes.

There is considerable symptom overlap among the sex chromosome aneuploid conditions that are trisomies, including KS, Trisomy X, and XYY. We say that the *phenotypes*, or observable behavioral and physical characteristics, of the three conditions are quite similar. Tall stature and long limbs characterize many, but not all, of these individuals. There may be subtle physical signs, such as *clinodactyly*, or curved little finger, which often signals a possible genetic disorder. Individuals with SCA are also slightly more likely to have birth defects, such as club foot, cleft palate, or genito-urinary malformations (including poorly developed kidneys). Many have early language delay and continue to experience some difficulties with expressive language throughout their lifetimes. They may also have fine and gross motor skill problems, tremors, or, infrequently, seizures. The rates of ADHD/ADD, anxiety and mood disorders, and other emotional difficulties are higher than in the general population. All of the trisomy conditions can result in lowered fertility, but this is considerably more important in KS compared to XYY and Trisomy X. Only those with KS consistently experience infertility and as well as significant co-morbid medical problems, many stemming from inadequate production of testosterone. A very small number of males with XYY will have testicular failure or infertility, and females with Trisomy X usually have normal puberty and fertility but can experience premature ovarian failure (early menopause).

This guide contains more information on KS than the other trisomy conditions for several reasons. KS is both more prevalent than either 47,XYY, or Trisomy X, and is diagnosed two to three times more frequently than 47,XYY, and Trisomy X, because there are more opportunities throughout the lifespan for diagnostic inquiry. There have also been many more research studies done and articles written about 47,XXY, than about the other two conditions. KS has a number of medical issues that need to be addressed, including the need for supplemental testosterone treatment and for fertility evaluation to determine if assisted reproductive technology may allow biological fatherhood. There is also more known about co-morbid health conditions that affect adults with KS compared to those with 47,XYY, or Trisomy X. An overview of the medical information is covered in this publication, as well.

In addition to KS, the guide does provide chapters devoted to specific information available at this time for both 47,XYY, and Trisomy X. It also provides additional information about variant forms of KS, characterized by 48 or 49 chromosomes, and some information for those females who have Tetrasomy X (48 chromosomes) or Pentasomy X (49 chromosomes). This chapter provides an overview of the genetics of extra X and Y chromosomes as well as discussing disclosure, which is common to all three conditions. The guide concludes with three chapters on psychosocial, educational and transition to adulthood issues, which affect all three conditions.

What is the cause of SCA and how commonly does it occur?

Sex chromosome aneuploid conditions are caused by random genetic errors in cell division. These errors can either occur when the egg or sperm are developing, which is called *meiosis,* or when the cells of the fertilized egg or embryo are dividing, which is called *mitosis.* In KS and Trisomy X, the error occurs because either 1) the egg or the sperm contained an extra X chromosome (a meiotic error), or 2) after fertilization, the fertilized egg or embryo (called a zygote) divided but one or both of the cells that resulted contained an extra X chromosome (a mitotic error). The error is the same in 47,XYY, but only sperm can transmit the extra Y copy as a result of meiosis error when the sperm is created. An error in mitosis, after fertilization, can also cause the cell divisions that result in an XYY cell with two Y chromosomes and an X chromosome.

When KS is caused by an egg or a sperm with an extra X chromosome, about half the time, the extra X was in the egg from the mother, and half the time, the extra X is in the sperm from the father. In Trisomy X, about 90 percent of the time, the extra X is in the egg from the mother. In women, increasing age leads to an increased risk of an additional X chromosome, but it is not nearly as pronounced as the association with Down's syndrome (Trisomy 21). This increased risk occurs because women are born with all the eggs (ova) that they will ever have, and more mistakes are possible during division when these eggs get older. An older father has much lower risk of having sperm with additional X or Y chromosomes as he ages, because sperm are newly formed continuously in a male.

The diagram of an error in meiosis (see page16) is an over-simplification of the multiple steps that occur in creating egg or sperm. It illustrates, however, how an error in either egg or sperm can result in a fertilized egg with an extra or a missing X or Y chromosome.

Meiosis errors resulting in sperm or eggs with extra X and/or Y chromosomes are not the result of any environmental or lifestyle factors. Some studies have looked at occupation, alcohol and tobacco use, and other factors in an attempt to determine behaviors and environmental causes that may be associated with additional risk of sex chromosome aneuploidy. None have been found. Sex chromosome aneuploidy is a random event, and it is not the "fault" of either parent.

Mitotic errors that occur after fertilization also are random events. If a mitotic error occurs as the fertilized egg or cells of the embryo divide,

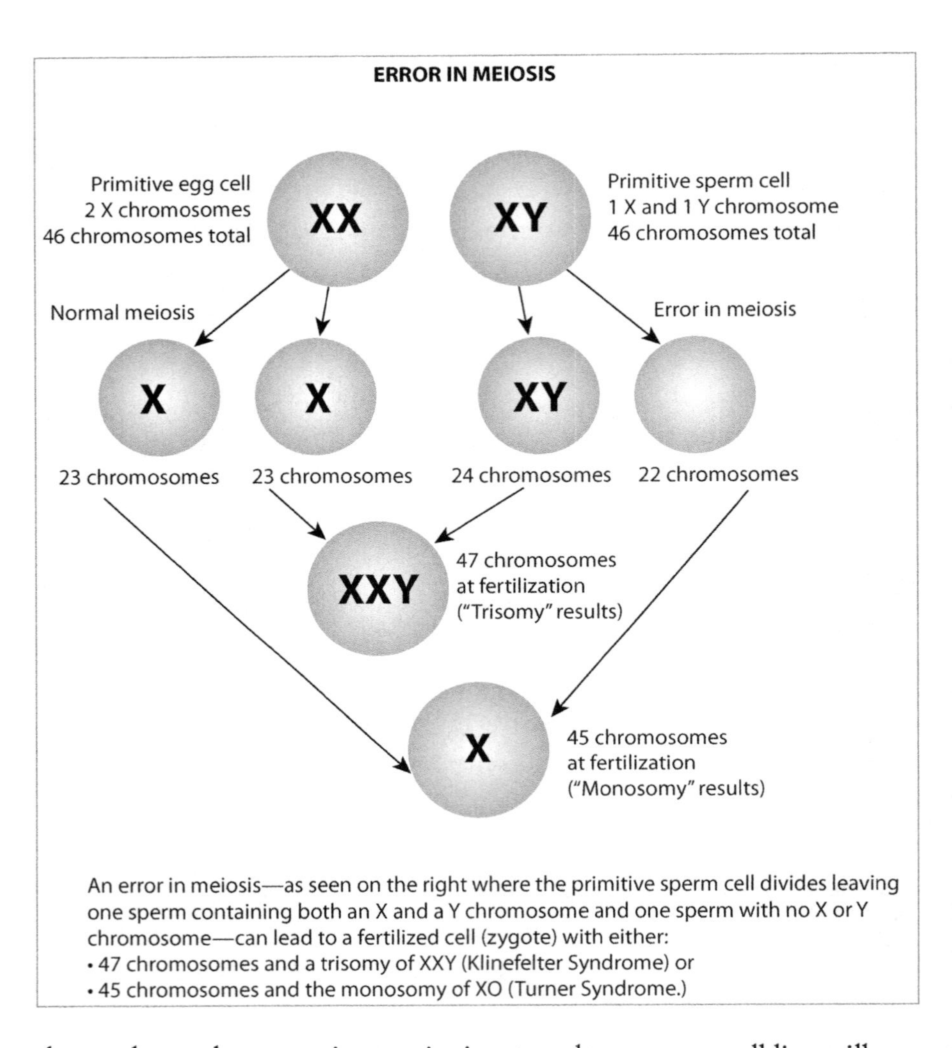

An error in meiosis—as seen on the right where the primitive sperm cell divides leaving one sperm containing both an X and a Y chromosome and one sperm with no X or Y chromosome—can lead to a fertilized cell (zygote) with either:
- 47 chromosomes and a trisomy of XXY (Klinefelter Syndrome) or
- 45 chromosomes and the monosomy of XO (Turner Syndrome.)

the result may be a mosaic genetic signature, because one cell line will have 47 chromosome with the trisomy (XXY, XYY, or XXX) and the other cell line will have 46 chromosomes with the XY or XX pair.

This diagram of mitosis is also a great over-simplification of the process of cell division. It illustrates, however, how a cell with the normal number of chromosomes can go through the process of division, in which the chromosomes double in number, and result in two new cells with errors in their number of X or Y chromosomes. This error can occur at any time after fertilization occurs.

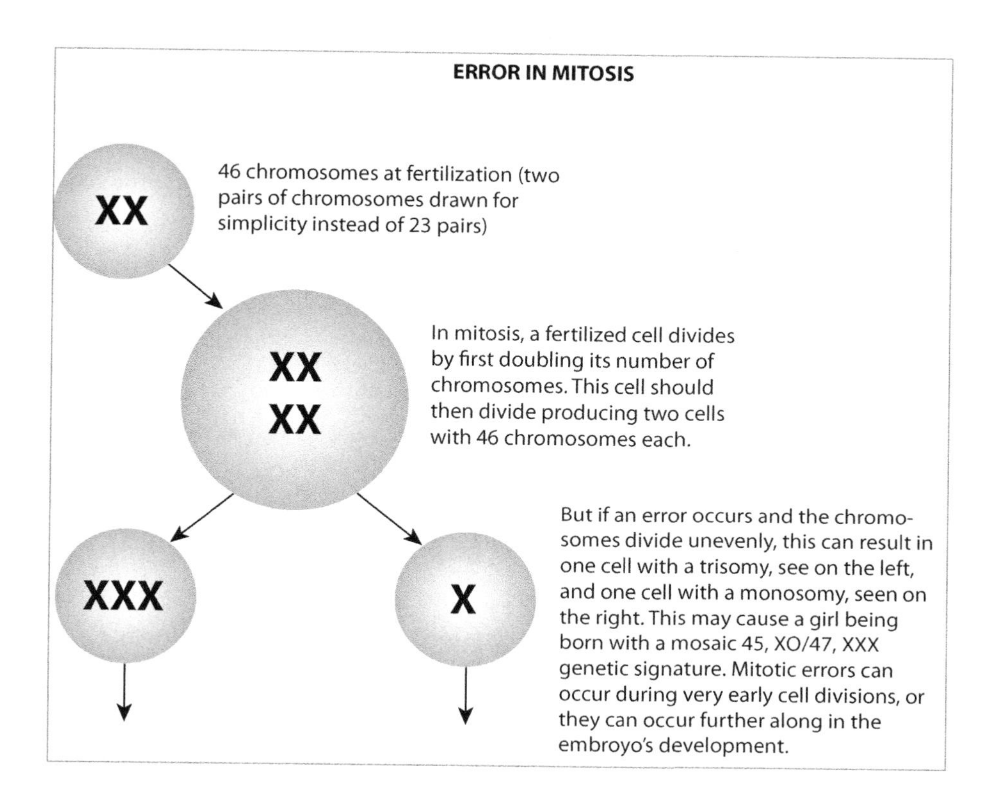

Although the SCA conditions that are being discussed are genetic disorders, they are not inherited disorders. The chance of recurrence of SCA in a family where one child has been born with SCA is less than 1 percent. And the chance that a man with KS who is fertile (which can be the case with mosaicism) will pass on KS to a pregnancy where he provides the sperm is also quite small. Similarly, adult men with 47,XYY, and adult women with 47,XXX, also have a very small chance of passing on the aneuploidy to offspring, although there are cases where this has occurred.

There have been studies showing a slightly increased risk of SCA of all types for pregnancies that have resulted from in vitro fertilization and especially from ICSI, intracytoplasmic sperm injection. This can be the case when a man with KS and his partner achieve a pregnancy using ICSI. For this reason, it may be recommended that pre-implantation genetic diagnosis of the embryos from a couple where the man has KS should be carried out prior to selecting the embryos to be placed in the woman's uterus. During this procedure called pre-implantation genetic diagnosis (PGD), one cell is removed from each embryo while they are still being cultured in the laboratory, and the cell examined to determine that if trisomy conditions exist. This allows for embryos with the typical number of chromosomes to be selected for implantation into the uterus.

We know that errors during meiosis and mitosis can result in the extra X and Y chromosomes that produce SCA. What about SCA, however, results in the phenotypic behavioral and physical characteristics that make up the syndromes of KS, 47,XYY, and Trisomy X? The question has not been well studied by researchers and we barely have a partial understanding. Determining the causes of the many symptoms that can make up the syndrome requires research into the genetic functioning of the extra chromosome(s).

It is speculated that the various symptoms that persons with SCA can exhibit occur because of the different levels of expression of genes from the extra X and/or Y chromosomes. In women, who normally have two X chromosomes, the genes on one X chromosome are usually "turned off" by the cell and that X chromosome is made into an inactive X chromosome. The inactive X chromosome shows up microscopically in the cell as a small structure called the Barr body. Some of the genes on the "inactive" X chromosome, however, have been shown to escape inactivation and continue to be expressed. These genes, then, are usually expressed as a "double-dose" in females with two X chromosomes. Many of the genes that escape inactivation are in areas of the sex chromosomes called the pseudoautosomal regions, which are regions on both the X and Y chromosome that govern pairing between the chromosomes during meiosis.

The genes in the pseudoautosomal regions of the X and Y chromosomes are similar (called homologous genes), and these genes are also usually expressed as a "double dose" in a typical male with one X and one Y chromosome. In the SCA conditions where there are extra X and/or Y chromosomes, the genes in the pseudoautosomal regions are being expressed in "triple dose" (for XXY, XXX and XYY) and in "quadruple dose" (for XXXY, XXYY, or XXXX), or more (for those with XXXXY and XXXXX). There are also some genes on the X chromosome outside of the pseudoautosomal region that may or may not be inactivated on the inactive X chromosome. In 47,XYY, or 48,XXYY, the additional Y chromosome is not partially inactivated, like extra X chromosomes. However, genes from the extra Y chromosome are also over-expressed. It is speculated that the more genes on the extra X or Y chromosome that are over-expressed, the more pronounced are the various symptoms associated with the SCA condition.

A good example of this is a gene called the SHOX gene which is located in the pseudoautosomal region of the sex chromosomes. The SHOX gene is important in bone growth, and typically SHOX is expressed in "double dose" from both the X chromosomes in a typical XX female or from the X and Y chromosome in a typical XY male. In all of the trisomy SCA conditions (XXY, XYY, XXX), the SHOX gene is expressed in "triple dose." This extra expression leads to extra growth of the long bones and the taller stature associated with these conditions. Interestingly, in Turner syndrome (the monosomy X condition where females only have on X chromosome), SHOX is only expressed from the single X chromosome. Turner syndrome is associated with short stature. Researchers believe that differences in the expression levels of other genes in the pseudoautosomal regions are responsible for the other features of the SCA conditions such as the speech delays and learning disabilities, however, they still do not know the specific genes that lead to these features.

The X chromosome, particularly, has an enormous number of genes, estimated to be as high as 2,000. The primary structure of genes is made up of DNA, or deoxyribonucleic acid. It contains two long strands of pairs of four nucleotides (molecules) represented by the letters, G, C, T and A. These strands form a spiral called a double helix that coils tightly enough that it can be seen under a microscope as 46 chromosomes, one of which is the X chromosome. Each gene contains the genetic information that, among other things, controls the precise structure of proteins produced in cells. A gene for making a protein essential for testosterone action in the body is contained on the Y chromosome. It contains repeating units of three nucleotides, CAG, that repeat themselves and the more repeats there are in the DNA, the LESS active testosterone may be. Thus, much research has focused on whether under-virilization in men is caused by this variation in DNA structure.

This sort of microscopic analysis needs to be carried out with hundreds of genes on the X and Y chromosomes in order to begin to understand both the differences that supernumerary sex chromosomes can produce, as well as the phenotypic variation among individuals with the same genetic signature. We are only just beginning to understand how the extra X and Y chromosomes and the additional genetic material affect individuals with SCA to produce the symptoms that can be associated with the conditions.

Overall, SCA occurs approximately once in every 400–500 live births. Taken as a whole, SCA is not really a rare disorder. The threshold for a rare disorder, according to the National Organization for Rare Disorders, NORD, is that the condition affects fewer than 200,000 persons in the United States. Klinefelter syndrome, which probably affects at least 300,000 individuals, exceeds the threshold alone. Add in XYY with 150,000 and Trisomy X with another 150,000, and the total number of individuals with SCA approaches 600,000. SCA deserves to be treated as a known genetic disorder that should be understood by health care professionals and considered when making differential diagnosis of developmental disabilities and other medical problems. Families and individuals affected by SCA, however, know that this is not at all the case.

Klinefelter syndrome, or 47,XXY, is the most common of the SCAs, occurring in 1 of 500 to 600 male births. Approximately 80 percent of these individuals have a non-mosaic karyotype with 47 chromosomes; 10 percent have a mosaic form of the condition; and another 10 percent have a variation of 48 chromosomes (48,XXXY, or 48,XXYY) or of 49 chromosomes (49,XXXXY). The KS variations with 48 chromosomes, however, are truly rare as are those with 49 chromosomes. It is estimated that 48,XXYY and 48,XXXY, occur in 1 in 17,000 to 1 in 50,000 male births. 49,XXXXY, is estimated to occur in 1 in 85,000 to 1 in 100,000 male births.

For KS, there is some data on prevalence within ethnic groups. In a recent newborn screening study to estimate rates of Fragile X, the methodology also detected XXY. For white males, the rate of XXY was found to be 1 in 602; for African-Americans, 1 in 549; for Hispanics, 1 in 1799; and for Asians, 1 in 282.

47,XYY is estimated to occur once in 1,000 male births, and 47,XXX, once in 1,000 female births. I was not able to find similar ethnic data such as exist for KS, for XYY, and XXX.

It has also been estimated that of pregnant women over 35 who undergo prenatal testing (amniocentesis or CVS, chorionic villus sampling) one quarter who have results of a chromosomal disorder will be told that the fetus has SCA. For woman over 35, the rate of SCA in pregnancies is 1 in 250. In a large study of 88,965 amniocenteses, the frequency of the chromosomal abnormally Trisomy 21 found during the second trimester for women less than 35 years was 1 in 572. This increased to 1 in 96 for women ages 35 and older.

For pregnant women age 39 or younger, the percentage of fetuses with SCA is actually greater than the percentage of fetuses having a diagnosis of Trisomy 21, or Down syndrome. Yet pre-testing counseling often emphasizes the risk of Down syndrome (because it is much better known) or other far more serious and disabling trisomy conditions.

Counselors have stated that the genetic results that they most fear are actually those of sex chromosome aneuploidy because there is relatively little information available for parents, and because the range of outcomes is so great. The chances of significant disability, however, are still quite low with the SCA trisomy conditions. It would seem as though counseling should emphasize this fact, rather than the small chance of a very negative outcome. Nonetheless, over 50 percent of those who receive a prenatal diagnosis of SCA still terminate the pregnancy. For those who are fortunate enough to encounter good quality counseling after a prenatal diagnosis of SCA, and for those who locate support from parents of children with SCA, termination rates are lower.

> *Our OB was encouraging. She had worked with Dr. Robinson in Denver and was knowledgeable and up to date on XXY. She offered to put me in touch with another XXY mom. The genetic counselor was absolutely neutral, and answered all questions based on research percentiles. She did inform us that 75% terminated, which she felt showed how ignorant many were about XXY/Klinefelter syndrome or because they feared the old yet still widely available information from the original prison studies.*

Several excellent articles exist that summarize functioning for these children as well as providing recommendations for care in early childhood. They are available online and should be provided to expectant parents and to their health care providers. (Please see Bibliography for citations and online access URLs.) Because the initial prenatal diagnosis is often given to parents by the obstetrician, it is imperative that accurate information be available to prenatal clinics.

Training programs to update obstetricians, midwives, and nursing and social work personnel in prenatal clinics should be easily available (perhaps as web-based continuing education) and should present current and unbiased data on SCA. There should also be easily readable pamphlets available in waiting areas to direct expectant parents to additional literature as well as to phone numbers and web addresses providing parent support.

Only ten per cent of cases of SCA are diagnosed prenatally, and this is generally limited to pregnant women who are 35 or over, or in women considered to be at risk of a more serious genetic problem. After the prenatal period, there is pronounced under-diagnosis. For KS, only 25 to 30 percent of males with the condition are ever properly diagnosed. For XYY and Trisomy X, the percentage of diagnosis over the life time is even lower, estimated at 12 percent and 10 percent, respectively. Children with SCA conditions with 48 and 49 chromosome variations are more likely to be diagnosed in infancy or toddlerhood because they have more significant presentations including dysmorphic facial and other physical features that lead doctors to recommend genetic testing. Even so, a substantial percentage of children with these variations go for years without being properly diagnosed.

Diagnosis of SCA, whether on a prenatal sample, or on a peripheral blood sample, is now routinely diagnosed by one of three different types of genetic tests: chromosome analysis (also called karyotyping), FISH testing or microarray testing.

A chromosome analysis or karyotype is created when special dyes are used to stain the chromosomes so that they can be photographed under a microscope and then arranged in pairs. This allows cytogenetic technicians to examine the chromosomes for structural as well as numerical abnormalities, and they can see and count the extra sex chromosomes in SCA.

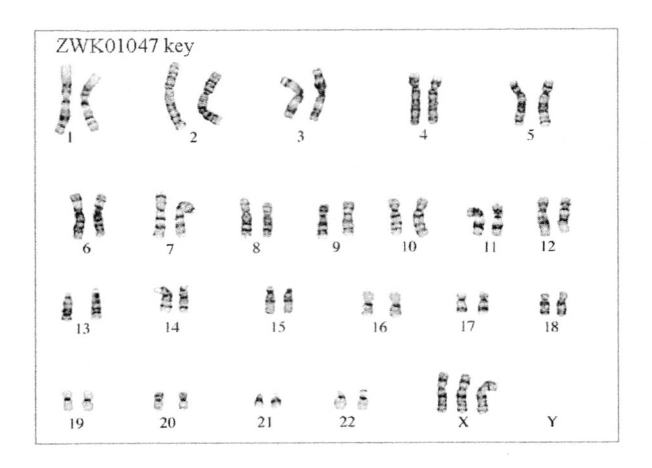

Karyotype of 47,XXX (Trisomy X)
[Used with permission of the Wisconsin State Laboratory of Hygiene, Board of Regents of the University of Wisconsin System.]

FISH stands for "fluorescence in situ hybridization" which is used to determine the number of copies in a cell of a specific small segment of DNA. In the lab, a "probe" is made by chemically modifying a segment of DNA and labeling it so that it looks fluorescent under a special microscope. Probes can find segments of DNA that indicate the presence of a trisomy condition. If SCA is diagnosed by FISH, it is often followed up by a karyotype or microarray test to look more carefully at all the chromosomes. Sometimes FISH is also done to look at a large number of cells to determine if there is mosaicism.

A microarray is the newest type of test available that is now identifying many cases of SCA. A microarray uses thousands of molecular probes to determine if there are any very small extra pieces (duplications) or missing pieces (deletions) of the chromosomes, and thus the results will also show if there are larger duplications such as the presence of an entire extra sex chromosome. Many doctors are now ordering microarray tests instead of karyotype tests when they suspect a genetic disorder because they are able to identify significantly more genetic abnormalities compared to a karyotype.

Prenatal genetic testing generally examines about 15 cells. It is recommended that genetic testing for SCA examine at least 20–30 cells to rule out mosaicism. If a child is diagnosed prenatally with SCA, genetic testing after birth should be done to confirm the diagnosis and to determine whether the child has any mosaicism. It should also be noted that this testing only determines the cell lines in peripheral blood samples. Even if there is no mosaicism in the blood cells, it is also possible that it can be present in other tissues, such as skin tissue or testicular tissue, although the chances are small.

If SCA is not detected prenatally, the chances of referral in childhood for genetic testing to explain a variety of physical and developmental delays are quite low. Unless the child has birth defects or pronounced developmental delay, the physical signs of SCA are quite subtle. They include hypotonia and sometimes clinodactyly (curved pinky finger). In boys with KS, there are sometimes physical signs including undescended testicles, micropenis or, less commonly, hypospadius, a penile abnormality where the opening for the urethra is either on top of or underneath the penis, rather than at the end. Speech delay is the most common symptom in children with SCA, and while doctors may refer the child for speech therapy they usually do not think it is severe enough to order genetic testing. Unfortunately, they do not often know enough about SCA conditions to suspect the diagnosis.

However, young children with the combination of symptoms including speech delay, low muscle tone and awkward coordination, and social skill deficits, will often trigger the suspicion of a possible autism spectrum disorder and referral to a developmental pediatrician or developmental center for further evaluation. Many children referred for autism evaluation do NOT meet the criteria for even mild autism, but a genetics referral for those with the constellation of symptoms that caused suspicion, however, would identify a number of children with SCA who currently go undiagnosed for years, if ever.

Increasing, a small but significant number of children who are identified with SCA first receive a diagnosis of Asperger syndrome or PDD-NOS (Pervasive Developmental Disorder-Not Otherwise Specified), both of which are mild forms of autism. We do know that the risk for autism spectrum disorders is increased in children with SCA, particularly for those with XYY and XXYY, although they are still usually mild forms of autism. The American Academy of Pediatrics recommends that any child with a diagnosis of an autism spectrum disorder also have genetic screening and testing. Unfortunately, this recommendation is not routinely followed, with cost being one concern. Karyotyping can be expensive, costing between $400 and $900, although it is usually covered by health insurance. Another concern seems to be parental reluctance to look at genetics as a possible cause of developmental problems.

> *Originally, our son was diagnosed with PDD-NOS [Pervasive Developmental Disorder—Not Otherwise Specified, a milder form of autism] by a child psychologist. An hour later, our son saw a developmental pediatrician who told the psychologist that she thought this might not be the complete diagnosis. She referred us for a karyotype to check for Fragile X. Three weeks later, we received the diagnosis of 47,XXY. The developmental pediatrician had a hunch, but wanted the test before telling us about her suspicions. We then saw a geneticist who read from an old medical journal. We were appalled by her lack of information, but because we had already found the Genetic.org list-serve and had done our own research, we felt it was a waste of time to see her.*

An additional factor is that many children with SCA are not referred earlier for genetic testing because doctors are not well educated on the SCA conditions and don't have a high level of suspicion for them. Many have a mistaken and outdated belief that SCA conditions are all associated with intellectual disability (previously called mental retardation.) Others don't know that early developmental delays are associated with SCA. If there is no intellectual disability (and this is rare in SCA), many pediatricians, primary care specialists, and even some specialists still believe there is no reason to look for an extra X or Y chromosome.

For girls with Trisomy X and boys with XYY, there are few other opportunities for genetic screening unless an astute doctor puts the developmental history together with learning disabilities, behavioral difficulties and perhaps tall stature or other physical features, and orders testing. With KS, however, adolescence is an excellent opportunity for the pediatrician or family doctor to detect small size testes, incomplete pubertal development, or gynecomastia (male breast development which occurs in 15–20% of males with KS.). While other signs of KS may be subtle, there is nothing subtle about abnormally small testes or failure to progress normally through puberty. The reason that the opportunity to diagnose KS is lost is that often doctors do not examine the genitals of teenage boys, and this clear sign is missed.

In adulthood, the most common reason for diagnosis of KS is infertility. This also must mean that most men do not have a thorough examination of their testicles, and only do so when there is a problem with conceiving a pregnancy or there is a urological problem. Doctors and the lay public are also becoming more aware of symptoms of testosterone deficiency: low energy, muscle weakness, decreased libido and sexual functioning. This is leading more men to seek evaluations of their testosterone levels which leads to increased diagnosis of KS, as well. For adults with either XXX or XYY, infertility is not seen often, so these adults do not have this opportunity for testing. An increasing number of adult women diagnosed with Trisomy X in adulthood, however, are tested and identified due to fertility problems. Fertility specialists are becoming aware of the possibility of Trisomy X in lowering fertility or in causing premature ovarian failure (premature menopause).

Now that we have the information, what do we do with it?

It used to be argued that there was no clear reason for identifying an individual with an extra X or Y chromosome, particularly because a significant number do not have severe symptoms. As late as 2000, I remember being told that since there were no universally agreed-on treatment recommendations, genetic information for parents would not be useful. In fact, there was the argument that this genetic information could cause needless worry for families. I suspect that the "worry" that professionals did not want to impose on families and individuals were the old myths about individuals with XXY and XYY who were thought to be at increased risk of criminal behavior.

My interviews with families and adults, and the information from the surveys that I collected, tell a completely different story about the usefulness of early and accurate diagnosis. Those who had a prenatal diagnosis are convinced that this helped them to identify and act on developmental delays, even if the delays were relatively mild. Had parents not had genetic information that their children could be at risk for speech or other developmental delays, they might not have accessed early intervention services. I did not encounter parents who told me that a prenatal diagnosis caused needless worry throughout the pregnancy. Once the diagnosis was made, information was obtained, and parents determined that they would continue the pregnancy, most went on to enjoy anticipating their babies' births.

The days immediately following a prenatal diagnosis, however, were often described to me as a "nightmare" of having to make a decision regarding the option for termination in a very short time period. Good information is scarce, and parents not infrequently are told by their obstetricians that the child will have such a significant level of disability that abortion is the only rational option. Even many geneticists and genetic counselors, while they are specifically trained not to be directive in their counseling, frequently can provide little in-depth information to parents that might be more reassuring. Not only are parents frightened and at a disadvantage in gathering information, but continuing the pregnancy may put them in a position of disregarding medical advice to terminate. It is not surprising that over half of all pregnancies where the fetus is diagnosed with SCA end in abortion.

> *Three obstetricians in a local hospital called a meeting to tell me and my husband that we have to terminate. We told them that we had informed ourselves about the disorder, and that we would not terminate. They told me that the baby would be a monster, or a hermaphrodite, and would have a very small penis, and that they had to refuse us their services. They said that they couldn't take responsibility for the result of this pregnancy. My next obstetrician, a famous Greek embryologist, told me that there is absolutely no reason to terminate a healthy XXY boy, and that all challenges of XXY are manageable.*

For many of us who have raised children with extra X or Y chromosomes, and for those adults who have SCA and yet have found that they can live quite successfully despite physical and psychological challenges, for a professional to actually recommend abortion seems inappropriate. There are never any guarantees when having children that they will be free of birth defects, or that they will be free of serious illness later in life. In the realm of difficulties that a child may face over his or her lifetime, most would argue that SCA does not rank among the most serious. In my opinion, and the opinions of many others who responded to the survey, abortion does seem to be a measure that is out of proportion to the small risk of severe developmental disability, or of severe difficulties developing later on, such as psychiatric disorders, that prove to be totally disabling.

That said, I have the perspective of a liberal Jewish feminist: I believe that abortion should be safe and legal when it is determined by a woman and her doctor that the pregnancy would result in a condition that could endanger her health or cause undue stress with which the family could not cope. With good quality, compassionate counseling, my husband and I determined that the risk of severe disability was remote, and that we could provide the resources to help a child with mild/moderate disabilities to live a good life. The vast majority of parents I have contacted who have faced a prenatal diagnosis of SCA agree with this statement.

It probably is the case that genetic counselors are so committed to unbiased counseling that provides the full range of options, including termination, that when a chromosomal disorder is diagnosed in a fetus, they feel obligated to present the option as equally valid with continuing the pregnancy. I respect this approach, but I also believe that families who receive such a prenatal diagnosis should receive counseling by professionals who have far more access to accurate and comprehensive information about SCA than is currently the case. The quality of the counseling and accuracy of the material presented plays an important role in whether or not parents decide to continue the pregnancy, and are appropriately prepared for the birth of a child who may have special needs.

Knowledge of possible symptoms that may affect their children can assist parents with obtaining anticipatory guidance for their children to help them meet developmental difficulties if they do occur. Over two-thirds of young children with SCA have speech delay, and a similar proportion have low muscle tone and motor skills that lag behind their peers. Parents who are aware of this risk need not wait to see if the delay resolves. These parents already have grounds to obtain early intervention services as soon as they become aware that developmental milestones are being missed.

In all SCA disorders, timely diagnosis can help to explain the reason for learning disabilities or behavioral and mental health problems. A clear genetic diagnosis paves the way for early intervention and special education services, as well as for government benefits and assistance programs including vocational services for adults who may need additional assistance to become established in a career. Learning of the diagnosis, as long as it is accompanied by accurate and compassionate counseling, provides parents and adults with the opportunity to be aware of some of the risks, without becoming needlessly worried.

> *My son's doctor noticed during a physical exam that his testes were small, and told us it could be a "rare" genetic disorder. He suggested we wait a year and see if they descended. I immediately researched "small testicles, genetic disorder" and found Klinefelter syndrome. My son's symptoms were "textbook." I immediately called the doctor and requested testing, because he was struggling in school and we needed to rule out this disorder. I explained the symptoms to my son, and the doctor agreed to testing.*

> *I first started feeling that I was different from other boys while in middle school. I was tall, skinny, and awkward. I developed a terrible acne problem. I had always struggled with concentrating and communicating clearly, and I had problems with relationships. My self-esteem was low. I had no energy and I felt like I was years behind everyone else my age. I was in counseling for anxiety and depression, trying to figure out what was wrong with me. When I finally got the diagnosis, I was greatly relieved to learn that there actually was a condition behind my problems, and that my concern about something being wrong was correct.*

For adolescents and for older adults, the reaction to the genetic diagnosis is most often that of relief, sometimes coupled with grief related to the fertility problems in KS. Adolescents and adults with any of the SCA conditions who have struggled with learning disabilities and puzzling emotional problems most often have told me that the diagnosis explained many things that they and their parents had been unable to reconcile, such as continual low grades despite normal intelligence and lots of effort in school. Those with KS can consult with an endocrinologist to determine if and when testosterone supplementation is indicated, and if it may help improve pubertal and muscular development, physical endurance, and mood, and help prevent osteoporosis. They can adjust to the need to explore assisted reproduction or adoption to build families. And they can take action to guard against co-morbid disorders and possible complications of KS, such as tooth decay, deep vein thrombosis, and Type 2 diabetes. For adults with XYY and Trisomy X, the small increased risk of passing SCA to offspring can be assessed by genetic counselors.

Disclosing the Diagnosis

The current accepted general opinion about **disclosure** (telling people about the diagnosis) is that genetic information is private and highly confidential and that the diagnosis should only be disclosed when it is useful to the child or adult to do so. Although many states and the Federal government in the United States have tried to eliminate the ability of insurance companies to discriminate against persons with genetic disorders in obtaining health or life insurance, this is one possible problem area. So is the possibility of employer discrimination against persons with extra X or Y chromosomes, due to lack of knowledge or information about the conditions. It is also quite possible that relatives or acquaintances who know of a person's diagnosis of SCA may go on-line and learn all sorts of myths about criminality and insanity, and apply them wrongfully to the person with SCA. There are many different opinions about disclosure, and here I present my own opinion and experience, as well as the opinions of a number of the survey respondents.

When there is a prenatal diagnosis, of course, parents will want and need support. They can best judge whether trusted friends or relatives can share this information with them, along with appropriate literature about the genetic condition. Prior to birth, with a prenatal diagnosis, it may not be necessary to share the information with anyone except the child's pediatrician. This position of waiting to see if any problems develop is a completely rational one, and is adopted by many expectant parents.

There are good reasons for disclosing the diagnosis to the pediatrician, however. Infants with extra X and Y chromosomes are at a small additional risk for birth defects, some subtle and some not so mild and innocuous. If the child immediately demonstrates hypotonia and difficulty latching on to nurse, parents will want to monitor his or her feeding and weight gain. Boys with 47,XXY (and sometimes boys with 47,XYY) can have small genitals or micropenis; a series of three shots of testosterone between the ages of two and five months may help to correct this.

Children diagnosed prenatally with SCA should also be monitored closely by their pediatricians for consistently meeting developmental milestones. Many parents find that infants with SCA develop completely normally until about nine or ten months. At that point, they may begin to show the impact of low muscle tone on upper body strength needed to sit alone and to pull up to furniture and cruise along. It is also at this point that a number of parents, particularly when there are older children in the household, begin to detect that the range of sounds and vocalizations is more limited than it should be. This can be the result of low muscle tone in the face and tongue, so that the more difficult sounds are not being made as often as they need to in order to progress on to speech.

A child who begins to show delay in meeting milestones should be referred for Early Intervention (EI) services. Parents need to advocate for their infants because while developmental delays are not inevitable, over half of these children have significant early speech delay, and about the same number also have fine and gross motor skill difficulties. Early intervention services vary a great deal from one state to another and from one country to another.

If there are shortages of openings for EI, then children with SCA may not qualify because their delays are less severe than those of children with conditions such as cerebral palsy or autism. The progress of children with SCA in EI can often be quite remarkable, so parents also may have to fight to have them continued in services, particularly once they turn three, when (in the United States) responsibility for services moves to the local school district.

When and if children need early intervention, special needs preschool, or other therapeutic services, parents can consider disclosing the diagnosis to relatives and to close and trusted friends, as well as to school teachers or early intervention therapists. There are a number of viewpoints and opinions about how specific to be. If the delay affects primarily speech, many parents prefer to simply explain that the child has a speech delay and is getting speech therapy services to address this. I am in favor of disclosing the diagnosis to the early intervention providers, to preschool education teachers, and to any other therapists that the child may have.

The reason that I disclosed John's diagnosis of KS is that I also wanted to educate them properly in what XXY is and is not. I always accompanied it with appropriate literature, and when I needed additional information, I wrote it myself. Many parents do not want to do this because they fear "labeling," but children who have speech delay, social deficits, and poor coordination will be labeled anyway. It seems more productive to have a correct label attached with a medical diagnosis, than a general and in-specific label of "slow," "clumsy," "clueless" or "lazy." Or worse, to have them attribute the delays to an understimulating home environment or to poor parenting.

Disclosure becomes more complex as the child becomes older and enters school. Many parents fear that if they disclose the full diagnosis, that any problems will be "blamed" on SCA, or that teachers will go online, see outdated and inaccurate information about criminal behavior or mental illness, and then begin to see these "characteristics" in the child. Some parents have also had poor experiences where the information in the record, which should be completely confidential, somehow made it out into the community. Neighbors then gossiped about the child, or a child with KS was asked by another child if he "really was a girl."

In the survey, I was told of geneticists and obstetricians who were adamant about not disclosing the diagnosis to anyone but the pediatrician. The problem is that two-thirds of these children require special education services. If the child simply has a label of "speech delay" or "learning disability," the child is required, in many states and countries, to show extreme low-functioning in those areas, often at the 10th percentile or less, in order to qualify for special education services. Children with SCA do not consistently perform at a level that is this low, and their delays are often more global, involving not only speech but also fine and gross motor skills, academic performance, and social functioning. If the diagnosis of SCA is used, the child may qualify for "other health impaired" or OHI, and the definition of disability may then be broader and less restrictively defined. Again, a parent who discloses this information to the school should accompany it with accurate and up-to-date information about the syndrome and about educational measures that can be effective in managing this child's behavior and learning in the classroom. This is then an exercise in educating the school system about these very common chromosomal conditions.

> *I want to weigh in on the subject of disclosing XYY. Our geneticist strongly advised us against telling anyone, including doctors, family, friends and school. However, we chose to let them know so that all could help our son and be on the lookout for any issues that might pop up. Our son was affected in many ways with speech delay, motor problems, immaturity, impulsivity and PDD. That said, we have never regretted our decision to disclose. The only thing that anyone knows about XYY is what we have told them. I usually mention the old studies in case anyone comes across them. We have been well-supported at both schools my son attended. I can't promise there won't be a bad experience with disclosure, but if no one ever talks about XYY, how will anyone ever learn about it and get accurate information?*

For those children with SCA who also have a diagnosis of ADHD or autism spectrum disorder, seizure disorder, or another co-morbid condition, it is up to the parent whether or not to disclose both conditions. During the 1990s, the possibility of using "autism spectrum disorder" opened to those of us who have children with SCA meeting the criteria for this diagnosis. It was admittedly easier to tell teachers and other parents that John had mild autism or PDD-NOS, without going into the details of the XXY diagnosis. Of course, it deprived them of an opportunity to learn about the relationship of SCA to autism spectrum disorders, ADHD, learning disabilities, and psychiatric disorders like depression.

I now disclose both disorders, because the presence of a developmental disability, mild autism, qualifies John to receive services from New York State's developmental disabilities agency. He lives in a supported apartment program for young adults with conditions such as high-functioning autism and mild cerebral palsy. New York State provides him with a life skills trainer and he has a job coach helping him to become established in a career. If he used only the Klinefelter syndrome diagnosis, he would not qualify unless he had intellectual disability, and his IQ is in the normal range.

Disclosure in high school, college, and other post-secondary programs will depend on the extent to which the condition impacts learning and the ability to work. If special vocational training and programming is sought, then the condition will need to be disclosed as a medical condition requiring accommodation. The same is true if a college student requires disability accommodations. If none of these accommodations are necessary, then the information can and should remain private. There is never any reason to disclose the condition on the job unless some accommodation must be sought under the Americans with Disabilities Act (ADA) or the Family and Medical Leave Act (FMLA).

The extent to which the information is disclosed to family and friends is often dependent on the child's functioning level, as well. If he or she is obviously delayed or has behavioral problems, then inclusion at family gatherings and social occasions is far more comfortable if the family has disclosed the condition, along with appropriate educational information and literature. It is not necessary, in the case of KS, to emphasize or even discuss potential infertility, except with very close friends or relatives. There have been remarkable advances in reproductive techniques in the past decade that now provide the possibility of biological fatherhood, and this can be conveyed, if parents wish. If there are behavioral, physical or speech implications, simply discuss those matters.

Once the child's diagnosis has been disclosed to anyone, however, it is also time to begin telling the child that he or she has an extra chromosome(s). This can begin with toddlerhood, if the child is receiving therapies. The disclosure should be nonchalant and can simply state that he or she is receiving speech therapy because "there are extra messages in each one of your cells" or "the genes helping your brain develop speech are a little different," for instance. A child should not be going to doctors and receiving therapies and special education services without understanding, at his individual level, that he has a condition that makes him unique and special, as we are all unique and special.

> *We made a special outing for the whole family when our son was 8. We told them about the extra Y chromosome and what it meant. Our son said that he already knew he was different. It was a very positive experience. I am glad we didn't wait any longer.*
>
> *My husband and I told her. We started by acknowledging that she had gone through quite a bit in terms of having speech and occupational therapy, and that she worked very hard in school. We asked her if she would like to know the reason for this, and she said, "Yes" so we told her in simple terms that her chromosomes tell her body and brain how to develop, and she has one extra X. We told her that this sometimes just happens, and that it is no ones fault and nothing to be ashamed of. We emphasized her many gifts and told her that we want to optimize her potential.*

When our son was 8, he asked us what was wrong and why he was so much taller than anyone else in his class. So we told him all the positive things that we knew, showed him a picture of his chromosomes, and he just thought that was cool. He tells people this is why he is tall.

There is no need to go into detail about possible lowered fertility or about adult health issues or the need for genetic counseling while the child is very young. It is much easier to begin introducing concerns regarding puberty (or testosterone therapy in boys with KS) if the child has "always" known about his genetic condition, at least as far back as he or she can remember. If parents wait until a child is 12 or 16 to disclose the diagnosis, it is probably too late. The child will already know that something about him is different, and I can almost guarantee that the child will be angry and resentful that the information was withheld, if they are told once they enter the wonderful and challenging years of adolescence.

In our survey, families disclosed the condition to relatives in 82 percent of families. For children in school, parents disclosed information about the condition to the school in 62 percent of cases.

With the start of puberty, however, the issue of normal development and reproduction becomes very important to these children. Schools do a notoriously poor job of providing accurate and candid information to middle-school children. If parents want their child to develop a healthy attitude toward sexuality and his or her body, the parent has the uncomfortable job of providing this education.

Some developmental disabilities centers do provide special education in sexuality and reproduction, and if you are lucky enough to have access to one of these programs, and if your child needs this approach, it is wise to take advantage of this. There are also some excellent guides to talking with children about sexuality and reproduction, and some are specifically written for children who may have learning or other disabilities.

For boys with KS, the discussions can be more complex and often occur over time. Focus of discussions should be limited to the problem that occasioned the diagnosis or the recognition that a problem may be related to KS. Boys need to understand that they are males in every genetic sense even though the extra X chromosome may modify the timing and extent of their development. Knowing their son has XXY prior to puberty allows parents, in consultation with physicians and therapists when appropriate, to become thoroughly informed about issues of puberty, virilization and future fertility.

Hormonal difficulties are quite rare in boys with 47,XYY, or in girls with Trisomy X, but a small percentage of these children will also need hormonal assistance in order to progress normally through puberty. Girls with Tetrasomy X (48,XXXX) and Pentasomy X (39,XXXXX) may require hormone treatment but this varies. It is at this point that parents need to tell children that these genetic issues are private and the business of no one else but a physician. Children should be warned against disclosing these issues to friends in middle, junior high, or high school because of the potential for teasing and bullying. They should also be given appropriate and accurate information about their chromosomal conditions, and told that if they should find outdated and untrue myths on-line, to bring it to the parent's attention but certainly not to believe it. Children need to understand that they do not have a "disease" or "illness," but rather that the difference in their bodies will mean that they may go for some additional checkups.

Any child diagnosed during adolescence or in early adulthood has to be told the diagnosis at the time it is made. In my opinion, every child has a right to know this information and it should never be withheld. It will not protect him or her to withhold information that parents and doctors already have. Children are intuitive, and they will suspect that something is wrong, and that their parents and doctors do not respect them enough to tell them.

For young adults and for adults, disclosure issues focus on what to tell good friends and in particular, what to tell people whom they are dating. Again, this is a matter for the adult's comfort level with confidential information. When dating, it probably is not necessary to disclose this information until the relationship becomes serious. Once both partners begin to plan for the long term, the partners begin disclosing confidential information, such as their medical history and any possible fertility problems. People who really love each other find ways around genetic challenges, such as SCA. It may be helpful to speak with a genetic counselor about any of these issues, or to have a consultation with a specialist in assisted reproduction if infertility is an issue of concern.

At this point, I believe that the risk of discrimination by employers and by insurers is still too great to make disclosure of extra chromosomal material routine. There may be instances where an employee must disclose this information to an employer. One instance might be the need to take medical leave and to obtain job protection by invoking the Family and Medical Leave Act. Another example would also the need to request a workplace accommodation under the Americans with Disabilities Act. Again, if necessary to disclose it should be accompanied by accurate information and resources to prevent discrimination and bias.

A Lifespan Approach to X and Y Aneuploid Chromosome Trisomies and their Variations

This guide contains lifespan information covering infancy, childhood, adolescence and adulthood for each of the supernumerary sex chromosome disorder groups: Klinefelter syndrome and variations; 47,XYY syndrome; and Trisomy X and the variations affecting females, Tetrasomy and Pentasomy X. The sections regarding Klinefelter syndrome are longer than those addressing 47,XYY, and Trisomy X, largely because there has been more research on KS than on the other conditions. There is also far more medical information on hormone supplementation, infertility treatment, and co-morbid health complications, for KS individuals which do not affect those with 47,XYY, or Trisomy X.

Most readers of this guide will be doing so because they themselves have the diagnosis, or a loved one, often a child, has been diagnosed with SCA. The most important thing to remember in reading through the guide's discussions of SCA through the lifespan and the impact of SCA on quality of life is that most affected individuals manifest some, but not all, of the possible symptoms and abnormalities associated with the diagnosis. In many people, SCA has a mild/moderate presentation. Responsive parenting, a good educational program, and competent medical care can help the individual to meet his challenges and achieve independence and a satisfactory quality of life. That is not to say that there are not persons with SCA who experience substantial disability throughout their lifetimes, but this is not the norm for the SCA trisomies. At the same time, it is necessary to be candid about the range of disability that is possible.

What this guide does do is to counter the myths about SCA that originated in the early studies of XXY and XYY in the population of inmates of prisons and mental hospitals. These biased samples were used to describe a population of persons who had criminal records, as well as high rates of intellectually disability (mental retardation) and severe mental illness. Unfortunately, these early descriptions of criminals and mental patients made it into medical texts commonly used by physicians even into recent years. And although XYY and XXY refer to male aneuploid conditions, many people associate Trisomy X with these two conditions, and then assume that the Trisomy X females are similarly affected. Despite considerable recent published research providing evidence to the contrary, misinformation continues to pervade material available on the internet, which ties SCA to intellectual disability and criminal behavior.

To the extent possible, each of the chapters on the SCA groups follows a life span model of what to expect in infants and preschoolers, school-aged children, adolescents and teens, and adults. The sections specific to each of the supernumerary X and Y chromosome groups are followed by three chapters that outline many of the commonalities shared by this group of disorders including psychosocial concerns and recommendations, educational strategies, and considerations to take in helping the young adult with SCA transition to adulthood.

Klinefelter Syndrome (47,XXY)

Throughout this chapter, as in the introductory chapter, 47,XXY, will be referred to as KS. Although a tiny minority of men with 47,XXY (probably one to two percent) escape any symptoms of Klinefelter syndrome, including hypogonadism and infertility, the great majority are affected by one or more symptoms. In any event, my conclusion is that a symptom-free adult with 47,XXY, or his parents or partner, would be unlikely to be reading this guide. For that reason, this guide uses the term "non-variant KS" to designate males with a genetic signature of 47,XXY, as opposed to those persons with the 48 or 49-chromosome variations. Those variations are covered in the section that follows the lifespan description of KS because the manifestations of the syndrome where there are 48 or 49 chromosomes can be more severe in terms of physical features and development.

Klinefelter syndrome was first described in 1942 by Dr. Harry Klinefelter and his coworkers at Boston's Massachusetts General Hospital who published a report about nine men who had sparse facial and body hair, enlarged breasts, small testes, and an inability to produce sperm. In the 1950s, when techniques had been developed to image the chromosomes, it was discovered that Klinefelter syndrome was caused by one or more additional X chromosomes.

During the 1970s, large-scale studies into the incidence of the condition (as well as related sex chromosome aneuploidy conditions including 47,XYY; 47,XXX, and variations involving 48 and 49 chromosomes) followed with several medical centers studying groups of children identified by newborn screening studies into young adulthood. Unfortunately, there had also been a series of studies of men with Klinefelter syndrome who were inmates of prisons and psychiatric hospitals, which provided highly biased samples leading to published conclusions that 47,XXY, (and 47,XYY) commonly leads to criminal behavior including sexual deviancy and pedophilia. Some studies also concluded that men with Klinefelter syndrome were likely to be mentally retarded (to have intellectual disability) or to have severe psychiatric disorders.

While the longitudinal studies provided excellent information about the development of children and young adults with SCA, the studies that are remembered and that more frequently made it into medical and psychology textbooks and common mythology were the sensational conclusions of studies of men in prisons and psychiatric hospitals. It has taken many years to begin undoing the harm of the early sensational study conclusions.

The almost universal finding in males with KS is testicular failure, which is the inability to make sufficient numbers of sperm and, in most, low testosterone levels. Becoming a father may be possible with complex and sometimes expensive treatment. Although most adolescents with KS enter puberty normally, and begin producing testosterone, puberty is often incomplete because the testes begin to fail in the mid-teens. While most men with KS have a penis of normal size, the testicles do not increase in size and are characteristically small. We also know that while many younger teens do produce viable sperm in the ejaculate through their mid-teens, this usually falls off precipitously early in puberty. This may not be true for boys with mosaic chromosome findings (XY/XXY). Sperm may be founds in the testes of adults with XXY and can be extracted for successful and normal pregnancies.

The other symptoms that characterize many males with Klinefelter syndrome include speech delay, low muscle tone and some difficulty with fine and gross motor skills, learning disabilities and social skill difficulties, including shyness and social withdrawal. Although boys with KS almost always develop functional language, expressive language, particularly written expression, may remain a challenge throughout life. Attention deficit disorder is more common in KS than in the general population, as are mood disorders and anxiety. Again, symptoms are highly variable from one individual to the next. While IQ may be slightly lower than that of siblings, on average about 15 points, intellectual disability (the preferred term for mental retardation) is rare, affecting less than 10 percent of those diagnosed with 47,XXY.

Although the condition of XX Male can be considered a variation of Klinefelter syndrome, it is not associated with the more severe physical or cognitive disorders of the 48 and 49 chromosome variations. An XX male has 46 chromosomes, as does an XY male. Rather than having the small Y chromosome, the part of its structure that determines male sexual development is attached to one of the X chromosomes so that he develops as a boy during pregnancy. It is also frequently the case that XX men, like those with 47,XXY, will have difficulties going through puberty, as well as learning disabilities and low testosterone.

In 80 percent of the cases of XX males, very detailed genetic study will determine that there is a tiny piece of the Y chromosome appended to an X that includes the sex determining genes of the Y chromosome. In 20 percent of the cases, no such sex determining genes seem to be present. In some of these cases, there may be ambiguous genitalia, and the person may have an intersex condition, but not always. This descriptive section on 47,XXY, is likely to be useful to those males who have a 46,XX, genetic signature because many of the features of KS will also apply to them.

Infants that have non-variant KS rarely look any different from any other newborns. There is a slightly increased risk of birth defects, most notably anomalies affecting the genitalia, such as hypospadias or micropenis. A few can have features such as clinodactyly (curved little finger) or hypertelorism, the medical term for wide-spaced eyes. There can be a variety of other birth defects, such as club foot or supernumerary digit or renal (kidney) defects, but the percentage of babies with significant birth defects is still very small.

For the parent with a prenatal diagnosis, the best recommendation is that her pediatrician should be fully informed regarding KS in an infant, and should conduct physical and developmental exams with that knowledge. Parents deserve to be able to anticipate their baby's birth and early infancy without undue worry about complications from KS, because there rarely are any. For parents who did not discover the extra X chromosome until later, it is unlikely that they missed clear signs of the condition, because in most cases there are not clear symptoms that lead a lay person to suspect a genetic condition.

For those parents who do have a prenatal diagnosis, the condition should be discussed with the pediatrician who has been chosen prior to the child's birth. After birth, if there is a question of determining whether there may be mosaicism, testing can be repeated, but testing on blood alone can never completely rule out mosaicism because another cell line may be present in other tissues of the body. It is not that important to continue to look for mosaicism in other tissues because the monitoring, treatments and follow-up will be the same for children with or without mosaicism. The child also should have a thorough physical examination for any signs of abnormality.

Physical abnormalities and other birth defects occur somewhat more frequently in children with KS than in the general population, although they are often subtle and may not be detected in a routine well child visit. Physical signs that may be present include *clinodactyly*, a curved little finger; *radio-ulnar synostosis*, fusion of the two bones of the forearm which leads to the inability to completely straighten out the elbows; and *pectus excavatum*, a depression in the sternum. Babies may have *micropenis*, or an abnormally small penis. Children with KS are also more likely to have undescended testicles, *cryptorchism*, or *hypospadias,* where the urethra opening is not at the end of the penis but rather on the upper or lower surface. There is also a slightly increased incidence of seizures, as well as an increased risk of other disorders such as a malformed kidney. The risk of significant birth defects is still low.

For those boys who seem to have an unusually small penis (micropenis) -and this will be the minority of babies with KS-parents need to be aware that there is a standard therapy for this condition. Whether or not the child has an extra X chromosome, an infant with an abnormally small penis should be referred to a pediatric endocrinologist or urologist for consultation on giving the child three shots of testosterone between the ages of two and five months. This will usually stimulate the penis to grow to and stay at a more normal size.

Some parents and some physicians believe that any boy with KS should have this series of shots and that it mimics the *mini-puberty,* or testosterone spike, that occurs in young boys at approximately the age of three months. It is, in fact, the only time during childhood prior to normal puberty when a young boy produces any significant level of testosterone at all. There has been speculation that the testosterone spike of early infancy, which may be missing in babies with KS, is also implicated in neurological and muscle development. Parents who are interested in this treatment should discuss this with their pediatricians or with a pediatric endocrinologist prior to the child's birth, if possible. Little research has been done on this testosterone spike, however, so there is no current data to support that treatment changes outcomes absent a diagnosis of micropenis.

Babies with KS need everything that all other babies need. They need lots of parental interaction and stimulation, including listening to their parents talking and encouraging them. Some parents and doctors believe that children with KS may be more prone to asthma and respiratory infections. This is complicated to determine, however, because both conditions are very common in children and there is no clear evidence one way or the other at this time. Babies can benefit from breast feeding, and mothers can provide extra health "insurance" for their sons by doing this. Due to the low muscle tone, some infants with KS have difficulty latching on and breastfeeding, and if this occurs, mothers should seek guidance by a lactation specialist if they want to continue breastfeeding. Pumped breast milk fed through a bottle is an alternative.

Babies, especially those at risk of motor problems, need lots of opportunities to move about freely, unconfined by walkers or strapped into seats, so that they can develop their muscles and motor skills.

Parents can dance with their babies to help them with balance. They can put them on their tummies when awake so that they push up and develop their upper bodies. Babies love games like "pat-a-cake" and songs like "itsy bitsy spider" that teach them hand motions. Parents can limit television and videos, especially if their children who are extra quiet and do not move around much. It doesn't hurt to watch the occasional show or DVD, but it is best if someone is interacting with the child while he views the program.

If developmental delays do surface, parents in the survey indicated that they were often not noticeable until late in the first twelve months of life or in the second year. For this reason, it is important that parents follow the regular schedule of pediatric visits and that the pediatrician perform regular developmental screening to determine that the child is meeting all milestones. Delays, as with most things related to KS, may be subtle and difficult to detect. For many children, speech and motor delays are caused by a combination of *dyspraxia,* in which the neurological processes that allow for motor planning to achieve movement and speech are not properly aligned, and *hypotonia,* which is low muscle tone. This may include slowness to walk, such as not taking the first independent steps until 15 or 16 months, which is still within the normal range but on the "slow" end. A limited range of vocalizations may be a feature of which parents slowly become aware. Parents may notice that the child doesn't point to draw their attention to something. The child may choose to sit for long periods of time, playing with only one toy and moving around very little. His balance may not be quite good enough to sit on the floor without making a "W" of his legs, indicating truncal or core weakness.

For parents who begin to feel uneasy about the child's development, a referral to a specialist such as a developmental pediatrician or a speech therapist skilled in children's speech disorders is in order. Most localities and counties in the United States have an early intervention program, funded as part of Federal Title V for children with special health care needs, which will provide free-of-charge evaluations as well as therapies up to age thirty-six months. Canada and Western Europe and other developed nations have similar programs.

> *Early diagnosis and aggressive, early therapy is extremely important. My child is a great example of what early therapy can do to benefit a child with his condition. After showing delays, he received physical therapy and speech twice a week for two years. The results and improvement were staggering.*
>
> *For parents receiving a prenatal diagnosis, it is critical to be educated about the wide range of degrees to which an individual may be affected by this genetic condition. Parents should also be given information about the expected age of developmental milestones. If they begin to see a lag, they should know how to contact Early Intervention and how to request an evaluation.*

Parents of babies with KS should be prepared for an early intervention evaluator with very little knowledge of sex chromosome aneuploidy. I recommend that they put together a packet of accurate information from legitimate websites and from this publication and provide the evaluator with copies. Be aware that many early intervention programs also require developmental delays that place the child significantly below the mean in order to approve free-of-charge services. If your child does not qualify for free-of-charge early intervention services, but you and your pediatrician still have concerns, you should be able to obtain services by getting a second opinion through a developmental pediatrician or other specialist. Your private medical insurance also may support therapeutic services, which can include physical and occupational therapy, and speech therapy.

Babies with KS may trigger the screening tools commonly used by pediatricians, such as the M-CHAT (Modified Checklist for Autism in Toddlers) or the ASQ (Ages and Stages Questionnaire), that are used to test for possible developmental disorders, such as autism or developmental delays. If your child does have concerns raised by one of these questionnaires, remember that these tests are just screening tools, which are showing that your child may be delayed in one or more areas. Abnormal results on these screening tests should result in referral to a developmental pediatrician or other specialist for further testing and diagnosis.

In our case, our son showed numerous delays and behaviors associated with what we now call *autism spectrum disorder.* Once he began receiving early intervention services, his development accelerated and he quickly made up time in meeting many milestones, rapidly acquiring speech where he had almost none, and progressing well with his motor development. In contrast to other children in his program with the diagnosis of classical autism, John made significant progress and has followed a completely different developmental trajectory, even though he retains a diagnosis of mild autism as an adult. Many parents of boys with KS have had the same experience when their children received services alongside children with diagnoses such as autism and intellectual disability.

It is frightening, however, as a parent to be told that ones child is developmentally delayed and needs such services. The American Academy of Pediatrics recommends that children with unexplained developmental delay or a diagnosis of any *pervasive developmental disorder* be referred for genetic testing. If pediatricians and parents actually followed through with this recommendation, children with sex chromosome aneuploidy would be diagnosed at a far higher rate than they are now.

It should be emphasized that children with KS tend to be exceptionally sweet babies, and that they are delightful children first, and babies with KS second. Mild delays do not stop you from loving your little boy and from finding his development absolutely awesome, even if it happens a few months behind schedule, and requires a bit of prodding from you and an early intervention therapist.

Preschool age is the time when children begin to explore outside of their homes and take an interest in socializing with other children. They go from engaging only in parallel play side by side with another child to interactive play. Whereas parents are enough of a universe for an infant, the preschool child becomes more interested in the world outside of him immediate family. Preschool is a time when your child can begin to go to see children's movies and puppet shows and when you can take him to a place like a children's museum, and he will remember the experience and want to return.

There are no specific health or developmental measures that parents need to take with preschool boys with KS. You and your pediatrician should continue to monitor his development in the speech and motor development areas. Any significant delays should be dealt with by referral to specialists for evaluation. Don't accept the comment that, "He is a boy. He'll grow out of it." Most boys with speech and other developmental delays don't just "grow out of it." Preschoolers need to begin seeing a dentist. Tell the dentist that your boy has KS. Many of these boys have thinner enamel than normal, and a large pulpy interior to molars, called *taurodontism.* Your dentist may want to seal his teeth against decay, or provide additional cleanings beyond the recommended two annual professional cleanings.

Preschool is also the time to help your child to develop healthy eating habits and an active lifestyle. A child with coordination difficulties will benefit from a variety of physical activities which make him feel good. For kids with KS, general development of upper body strength is critical to developing good writing and keyboarding skills. Ask a fitness expert to give you and your son an age-appropriate workout program to do at home that concentrates on strength training for both of you. Walk, ride bikes (he may need training wheels for some time), go horseback riding, swim, play miniature golf, and climb on play equipment together. You can also try sports such as T-ball but allow your son to guide you about what he feels comfortable in doing. If he is uncomfortable with sports "pressure," he may be too young for you to insist that he follow through with a season of team sports.

Many parents of boys with KS can benefit from a brief consultation with a physical therapist to design an exercise program that will address the mild difficulties caused by somewhat weak upper body and trunk muscles. This exercise program can be carried out at home by the parents using inexpensive equipment such as an exercise ball, elastic bands, and simple equipment to promote balance.

Boys with KS may not develop adequate bone density unless they have enough calcium and vitamin D in their diets. They also are prone to tooth decay, and later in life, to collecting fat around the middle. For that reason, sugary sodas and fruit juices should be limited, and boys encouraged to drink low-fat milk and to eat other dairy products, as well as a high-protein diet.

Because of low muscle tone in their stomachs and abdomens, boys with KS should be encouraged to eat complex carbohydrates with adequate fiber to counteract the constipation that many experience. Children who are bothered by constipation and pain may develop a vicious cycle of holding back bowel movements, causing "staining" and then accidents from loss of control. A child having lots of difficulty with constipation can have a mild stool softener recommended by a doctor. Increasing the child's intake of fruits and vegetables can also help.

Developmentally, some boys with KS are not ready to toilet-train completely by age three. They may be urine-trained during the day but be unable to keep dry consistently at night. Bedwetting after age seven is commonly reported by parents of boys with KS. Remember that this is most likely a result of developmental and maturation issues, and that the boy is not doing this in any willful manner. Disposable "Pull-ups" can help him get through this stage along with waterproof sheets and patience. Don't lose your temper at him, regardless of the frustration that you feel at having to change bedding. Most boys with KS manage to stay dry at night by age ten.

To get your son ready for school when kindergarten comes around, the most important thing that you can do is to read to him and give him lots of opportunities to listen to music, draw and paint, and travel to parks, museums, science exhibits and other places where he can learn about his world. Take him on nature walks, give him responsibility for a pet, introduce him to the planets and outer space, and let him ride on a variety of modes of transportation- planes, trains, buses, hay rides. Stretch his mind by taking him to experience a zoo, a farm, and an arboretum or conservatory. Make sure that he gets to spend time with grandparents and others who love him and will help him to develop a good strong sense of self-esteem.

> *Our son is a happy, joyful child. He is loving, kind, polite and even at age 4 says, "Please," "Thank you," "God bless you." He is sweet and sensitive and loves to play creative games as well as with his trucks and trains. He always asks for a "hug and kiss" before Mommy leaves for work.*

It is not possible to generalize about how KS may affect a preschool boy behaviorally. Although many of these boys are described as quiet, sensitive, and somewhat withdrawn socially, boys with KS display a complete range of personality types. However, many of the parents do describe some behaviors that can be more challenging than they have experienced with their sons' siblings. Some of the behaviors that parents may experience may appear to be a bit immature, with their KS sons holding onto "comfort" toys and objects, such as crib blankets and stuffed animals, longer than their siblings did. They may suck their thumbs later than sibs, be "clingier" with parents, and they may appear to be quick to show frustration, often in the form of temper tantrums or crying episodes. While frustration temper tantrums and crying tend to taper off after toddlerhood, some parents of boys with KS report that these behaviors continue well into the preschool and elementary school ages.

What parents may be seeing are children who are slightly delayed, in that they walk late, at 15 to 18 months, and while their receptive language is normal for their age, their expressive language lags rather significantly. They may also lack the motor skills that their peers have, and in general perform at a level that is "behind" that of children of a similar age. In preschool classes, boys with KS may lack both the verbal and social skills to feel completely comfortable. As a parent, you need to make certain that you are not pushing him into situations for which he does not yet have the coping skills. At the same time, it is good to expand his social experiences and to encourage play but it is also necessary to recognize when he may be in a position where he becomes so uncomfortable that it becomes an aversive event. While your son is unlikely to be as impaired as a child with intellectual disability or one who clearly falls onto the autism spectrum, he may have mild delays in a number of areas of communication and motor skills.

Coping with tantrums and meltdowns is something that many parents of boys with KS, and with all SCAs, report as being the most difficult part of parenting these children. Some of the difficulty appears to stem from immaturity compared with peers. Parents also report that many of these boys are acutely sensitive to loud noises and to overwhelming experiences, such as crowded sports stadiums. Many of them cannot tolerate labels in their clothing, and they are very picky about the "feeling" of socks and other clothing that touches their skin. They report that their children have difficulty adapting to rapid change in routines, and that their children have over-the-top reactions to situations that scare them, like loud trains coming into stations, or barking dogs.

When a child moves from the early intervention to preschool services, families of children with milder disorders, such as KS, often find that they are encouraged to decrease service levels, or to abandon services altogether. The problem is that with children with KS, the collective impact of mild/moderate delays in multiple areas—speech, motor skills, and social skills—can impact the child quite negatively once school starts. It is important to minimize the child's delays before he reaches kindergarten. For that reason, a tenacious approach to obtaining therapeutic services is warranted in most cases. Many parents opt for developmental or neuropsychological testing by a private specialist in order to have the data available to argue for continuation of services by the school district. Parents whose health insurance will cover therapies can augment the services provided by the school district.

Concerns regarding the **school age** boy with KS generally center on helping to ensure that he succeeds in school academically and that he is able to make friends. Elementary school in the United States and Canada generally runs from kindergarten to fourth or fifth grade in districts with middle schools, to sixth grade in districts with junior high schools. There are numerous exceptions to these grade groupings. In general, children get their reading and math foundations in grades K-3, so primary school or elementary school is very important. Children also establish themselves socially with other children on the playground and in after-school activities.

Kindergarten, once half a day of play, now usually encompasses a four and one-half to five hour day with academic pressures that you may not have experienced as a child. Be certain that your son is ready to sit at a table and to perform focused tasks involving numbers and letters, and even reading. Many parents hold back any child, especially a boy, born in the summer or later, to allow him to have an additional year of preschool before beginning kindergarten. Although this is a controversial practice, many parents reported that their sons with KS really benefitted from that additional year of emotional and physical maturation.

Children who will be enrolled in kindergarten are usually screened in the spring before their kindergarten year. If your child has not had any special services as a preschooler, he will be tested for reading and math readiness, and will be screened developmentally for social readiness. The reason that I am discussing learning disabilities in this section is that our survey found that nearly 75 percent of boys with KS did require some special education services in school, from simple accommodations like extra time on testing to speech therapy, resource room or special reading programs, occupational therapy, and even self-contained classrooms. This finding is consistent with the findings of the previous prospective follow-up studies in KS, as well.

In addition to academic concerns, enrollment in elementary school brings up a whole new world of social concerns, from getting along at lunchtime to playing at recess and having friends over after school. He should have a variety of opportunities to socialize, but make certain that the opportunities include activities that he likes, and that the social setting is one in which he feels comfortable. If you detect that he is beginning to struggle socially, it is worth trying to determine what may be causing this. Boys who are comparatively immature may not have the verbal skills or social skills to interact confidently in a given situation. If this is the case, find a speech therapist or behavioral therapist who offers social skills classes and activities that can help him to develop these skills in a supportive atmosphere. Socializing in an inclusive setting where there are both typically developing children as well as children with mild learning and other disabilities can provide him with a setting in which he feels comfortable without being labeled as "different." The key to helping him succeed is to acknowledge that he may have mild deficits that can be addressed effectively, but to be upbeat and matter-of-fact about his learning or social differences.

> *Our son is caring and compassionate, reads avidly and is creative in building things. He is in the 90th percentile in visual-spatial perception. He often "sees" things that others don't. An example: "Mom, that cloud looks like Idaho!"*
>
> *My son only received additional services besides speech therapy because he was diagnosed with PDD-NOS (a milder form of autism) but otherwise did not qualify for special services with the diagnosis of Klinefelter syndrome alone. Once he started to receive additional services, he has seemed much more comfortable with school and more happy in general.*

If your child begins to struggle some in primary grades, it is especially important to let him know that this is not his fault, and that it has nothing to do with being lazy. At ages six, seven or eight, you can begin telling him in a very general way that his body was born with some minor differences, which is why he has had speech therapy, for instance, or he goes to a special reading class. It isn't necessary at this point to give him the difficult-to-pronounce diagnosis or to provide lots of detail. I told my son that he had extra "messages" in his cells that made it a bit difficult for him to talk when little, or to write by hand once in school.

By the time that he is nine or ten, he should have seen a pediatric endocrinologist to begin monitoring of progress into and through puberty. It is best that this not be the first time that he has heard that he has a "difference" in his body.

There are no specific medical measures to take in elementary school. You may notice that his growth in height accelerates somewhat after age six, and that his body takes on a "leggy" look. Many boys with KS do become tall for their age, and they develop long limbs. Often, their leg length from waist to foot will exceed the length between seat and top of the head. Their arm span, which should be roughly equal to height, often exceeds it. This is characteristic of KS.

His joints may be hyper-flexible, and he may continue to have poor balance. You can help counter this physical awkwardness by continuing to encourage activities that build upper-body strength and by being physically active with him. Karate, swimming, golf, hiking, fishing, cycling, skiing, kayaking or sailing, and weight-training are among the activities that he is likely to be able to do without fear of doing poorly in competition with others. If he likes team sports, by all means have him participate, but don't force him to do so if he is reluctant.

Continue to encourage a good diet that includes plenty of calcium. Fiber continues to be important for these children. If he does not like to eat fruits and vegetables, then blend them into smoothies, spaghetti and pizza sauce, home-made muffins, etc. Picky eaters should get a multivitamin, but megadoses of anything are unwise unless prescribed by a physician. Some doctors encourage fish oil that provides omega-3 fatty acids as a means of improving brain function and attention, decreasing anxiety and depression, and improving cardiovascular health. There is some research to support this. Check with your pediatrician about dosage and recommended sources before starting this.

You also need to encourage him to take good care of his teeth because he may be more prone to decay. Some parents will have their sons' teeth cleaned every three months, rather than every six months, to minimize decay and catch it early. To protect his teeth, don't allow sugary soda. Also realize that diet soda can reduce absorption of calcium, so it is good to limit diet soda to one a day, and make sure that he drinks low-fat milk or eats yogurt and low-fat cheese.

Another thing that I learned from the survey is how prevalent attention deficit disorder and anxiety/depression are among school-age children with KS. Thirty percent of men and boys with non-variant KS have been diagnosed with ADHD and nearly 50 percent with depression and anxiety. ADHD is likely to show up first in elementary school, and in KS boys, it may be the non-hyperactive inattentive presentation that makes concentration in school so difficult. Some boys also show impulsivity, in that they take actions without thinking of the consequences, like throwing things in class or hitting a sibling when irritated.

There are measures that can be taken to diminish ADHD in the classroom, like having the child sit near the front of the class, and placing him in a setting with a lower enrollment. A combination of medication and behavioral measures will work best if the ADHD is compromising home life and school performance. Children with KS who are suspected of having ADHD should be seen and treated by a developmental pediatrician or a child psychiatrist who can use appropriate measures (such as Connors scales) to make a definitive diagnosis and be able to monitor both effectiveness and any side effects.

Depression and anxiety can stem from a variety of causes, including social insecurity or the frustration of not doing well in school. Depression and anxiety can also have no clear cause and be the result of biochemical imbalances or structural problems in the brain. In boys with KS who develop anxiety and/or depression in elementary school, the cause is probably a combination or environmental factors as well as brain differences directly related to the extra chromosome. In elementary school children, anxiety and depression will often not present in the same manner as these problems do with adults. Children may cry and feel sad, but just as often, anxiety and depression can present as aggressive behavior, with the child trashing his bedroom and hitting other children or his family members. The psychiatric difficulties that can be co-morbid with KS and other SCAs are among the most difficult for families. After John's prenatal diagnosis, I had expected learning disabilities but I had not expected the severe depression that periodically emerged in my son throughout his school years. If you are seeing these symptoms then it is important to consult with a psychologist and a physician to receive appropriate diagnoses and to develop a treatment plan which may include behavioral therapies and possibly medication.

Adolescence in the boy with KS brings with it puberty and, frequently, the need to begin treatment with testosterone (sometimes just indicated as "T") if puberty does not progress normally. Puberty is characterized by the replacement of soft, straight hair over parts of the body by coarse, curly, often dark hair. This begins with hair under the arms—called adrenarche because it is thought to be due to small amounts of testosterone produced by the adrenal gland that makes cortisone. At the same time, the first event of the reproductive system is the secretion of a pituitary hormone, LH (luteinizing hormone). Initially, it is secreted only at night and testosterone levels during the day are low. However, prior to obvious virilization, this nocturnal testosterone causes cells in the testis to grow. Thus, an increase in testicular size is usually the first sign that a boy is entering puberty, although this change is frequently not noted by physicians, parents or the boy himself. This growth is the testis is limited in boys with KS.

Eventually, LH is secreted 24 hours a day, resulting in the beginning of body hair growth, an increase in height, changes in voice, muscle definition and growth of the penis and scrotum. During early puberty, both XY and XXY boys may exhibit some increase in breast tissue and/or fat. In most XY boys, this "gynecomastia" resolves within a year. It may be more prominent and persist in XXY boys.

At the same time, another pituitary hormone, FSH (follicle stimulating hormone), also begins to stimulate the multiplication of "germ cells," those cells that produce sperm. This causes further growth of the testes and fullness of the scrotum. In adult men, 80–90% of the volume of the testis is made up of cells that make sperm and only 10–15% is made up of testosterone producing cells. The growth of the testes is limited in boys who do not have normal numbers of germ cells and in boys who lack pituitary hormones, LH and FSH.

Current best practice for managing the adolescent boy with KS includes determining when puberty has started, and monitoring the boy's progress. This consists of a physical examination to assess general overall health. The endocrinologist will note development of underarm and pubic hair, examine the testicles, and measure penile length to determine stage of puberty, known as "Tanner stage." The doctor will also look at body proportions and note any obvious physical abnormalities. A hand X-ray may be done to measure bone age, and the doctor may send the boy for blood work to measure testosterone levels and gonadotropins, LH and FSH, as measures of the extent to which puberty has begun, if at all, and whether there is evidence that the testes have begun to fail.

Secretion of LH and FSH by the pituitary is controlled by a part of the brain called the hypothalamus. As the testes grow, they secrete testosterone and a protein called inhibin that signals the brain that the testes are working normally. If the testes cannot make enough testosterone, the brain causes the pituitary to make increased amounts of LH, measurable by a blood test. FSH stimulates the Sertoli cells to increase germ cells and sperm. If there is a deficiency in the number of germ cells, as there may be in KS, FSH levels will continue to rise in an effort to correct the deficiency. In addition, a deficiency in the number of germ cells prevents the cells that make testosterone from responding to LH and LH levels rise. The hormonal signs that the testes are not working normally can be determined by blood tests.

It is likely that boys with KS have a reduced number of Sertoli and germ cells, although the timing and extent of this deficiency varies and is not well understood. However, the growth of the testes in early puberty may be limited and eventually the testosterone production may be reduced, slowing the external signs of progression of puberty. When this happens, LH and FSH may rise to abnormally high levels. It is not know whether these high levels actually cause further damage or only reflect the progressive loss of the ability of cells in the testis to respond. High LH levels may increase estrogen production by the testes and increase the amount and duration of breast growth seen in XY boys.

It is not precisely known how many sperm producing cells, Sertoli and germ cells, are in the testes of boys with KS as they enter puberty. If there is progressive loss of these cells during puberty, we do not know what causes this to happen nor do we know the timing and extent of the loss. We do know that many adult men with KS continue to produce small numbers of normal sperm that can be successful retrieved for pregnancy and birth of healthy XX and XY children. We also know that some men with KS make sufficient amounts of testosterone despite high levels of LH and FSH. Further research is need to determine the treatment plan that will maximize the chances of fertility.

Further research is also needed to know when and how much testosterone should be given to supplement completion of pubertal changes and/or to preserve germ cells. It is known that some boys with KS produce sperm that may be cryopreserved for possible future pregnancy. Opinions differ regarding the timing and type of treatment. The judgment of pediatric and adult endocrinologists, fertility experts and urologists most familiar with these treatments should be sought.

For boys who have not been diagnosed prior to puberty, and for boys whose parents and physicians are not aware of the importance of helping along stalled puberty with testosterone, the teen years can become a time of insecurity focused on their bodies' failure to become more masculine. Men who only later were diagnosed have expressed their anguish over watching friends and classmates mature while they failed to develop facial hair, adult musculature and mature genitalia. The survey included numerous stories of men who knew that something was wrong, and that something was different about not only their bodies but also with their brains.

> *I was 17, the spring of my junior year in high school. My doctor called in a specialist to meet with us at the local hospital. The specialist did a physical exam and several measurements, and was telling me what each measurement meant. After the physical, he sat me down with my parents, and explained clearly about Klinefelter syndrome. He told me I would start on testosterone immediately. He was very clear in his explanations and answers to our questions, and he was very caring. I will always remember what a huge wave of relief came over me when he finally explained that the condition I had was not normal and could be treated!*

We now know that hypogonadal men can suffer from depression and irritability, that they lack stamina and feel fatigued, and that they often lack sexual interest. Imagine the adolescent who not only feels insecure about his immature-looking body, but also suffers from depression and fatigue, and wonders why he has little interest in sex when all of his peers seem obsessed with it. Adolescents can express this confusion and their anxieties by withdrawing from family and friends, by explosive acting out or by getting involved in substance abuse or impulsive acts, such as shoplifting.

Beginning at about age nine, a boy with KS should begin seeing a pediatric endocrinologist or other specialist who is familiar with the most recent recommendations for monitoring puberty and for treating KS. If no local physician has this level of knowledge, it is critical that parents travel to a university-based consultant, or other specialist, who can advise the child's local pediatrician or endocrinologist on managing treatment.

In all boys, a fraction of circulating testosterone is normally converted to estrogen-like hormones. The fraction of testosterone that is converted to estradiol is high in early puberty when testosterone levels are low and, as testosterone rises, the fractional conversion decreases. This is why the breast enlargement that many boys experience in early puberty resolves. There are two reasons why XXY boys may have high estrogens. First, if the testosterone rise is slow, the enzyme that converts testosterone to estradiol is not suppressed sufficiently. Second, if LH levels rise in mid to late puberty in an attempt to increase testosterone, this "hyperstimulation" causes more estradiol production by the testis. While a boy may have a low-normal level of testosterone, he may also have too high a level of estrogen and persistence of breast enlargement.

The goal of testosterone supplementation in an adolescent with XXY is to promote development of secondary sexual characteristics, such as growth of a beard and body hair. It also helps to allow boys to develop male body fat distribution, muscle mass, and bone density. There is a great deal of variation in the amount of estrogen made by KS boys. If puberty slows and testosterone levels are below normal, testosterone supplementation to restore normal levels will reduce estrogen levels and may prevent further breast enlargement, if present. Supplemental testosterone is also reported to help to reduce fatigue in adolescents, as well as having a positive impact on attention, behavior, mood, and academic performance.

Testosterone treatment is usually started in early to mid-puberty when LH and FSH begin to rise, which indicates the beginning of testicular failure. Hormone doses at initiation of therapy are quite low and are increased slowly. There is some disagreement among professionals about the route of supplemental T for an adolescent: gel or injection. Because small packets or each pump of gel distribute more testosterone than has been studied for the induction of puberty, there are many physicians who believe that a boy should start with monthly injections of 50 to 75 mg of one of the long-acting preparations, testosterone enanthate or testosterone cypionate. This can increase slowly until an adolescent in mid-puberty is receiving 100 mg twice monthly, at which point he can switch to 1.25 mg to 2.5 mg of gel per day. Other physicians initiate therapy using a small amount of gel daily in order to avoid the very blood high levels of T that are present immediately following an injection. There is some evidence that the very high level of testosterone produced by just after an injection can choke off sperm production. If the boy and his parents are interested in cryo-preservation of sperm for later use in ICSI, then they may want to use gel.

> *We told him immediately because he was 16 and we were heading to the endocrinologist to begin testosterone therapy. His levels were extremely low at 250, and he was weak and exhausted and had no stamina for any activity. He took the diagnosis well. He already knew he was infertile because he had been listening in biology class! In a way it was a relief to him to know why he felt a bit different from his brothers and his peers.*

Parents, their son, and the doctor must weigh the pros and cons of using gel and using injections. They must consider the dislike of adolescents for needles as well as the known tendency of adolescents to be spotty in their compliance with a routine requiring daily application of gel. Some families contend that while the gel provides a very even level of testosterone, it does not seem to have as beneficial an impact on reducing fatigue and regulating behavior as injected testosterone. No studies exist at this time comparing the two methods.

There are three possible approaches to fertility in persons with KS. First, in rare cases, men with mosaicism XX/XXY, sperm production may be sufficient for pregnancy without special treatment. Second, some boys with XXY may produce sufficient sperm in early puberty to "freeze" (cryopreserve in liquid nitrogen by a licensed sperm bank) sperm. Although sperm have been observed in KS boys in early puberty and can be retrieved from seminal fluid after masturbation, the normalcy of these sperm and their survival with prolonged cryopreservation has not been established. The cost of prolonged storage varies considerably. Some developmental psychologists have expressed concern about the possible impact of these procedures upon boys at this stage of sexual development. A third alternative is to seek professional help from in vitro fertilization (IVF) experts at the time a KS adult desires a pregnancy. There is a high rate of sperm retrieval by testicular biopsy from KS adults and successful pregnancies achieved by IVF units skilled in intracytoplasmic sperm injection (injection of sperm into eggs to achieve fertilization). Basic science reproductive research may be successful in the future in successfully producing sperm from germ cells in the test tube. Long term clinical studies are required to establish the best approach to fertility in KS men.

In order to work most effectively with the doctor, parents need to explain KS to their son as clearly as possible. It may help to show the boy a graphic of the chromosomes in the cell and to explain that the extra X has nothing to do with sexuality or "maleness"; it is simply an extra bit of genetic material that may have something to do with learning and speech disabilities, if he has experienced any. Explain that KS may also make it necessary for him to take supplemental hormone to complete his masculine development. Explain that he is in no way "part girl" and that this condition is actually rather common.

It is best to do the simple explanation first just before puberty begins, and to let him become comfortable with the knowledge before going on into the complexities of infertility, which may be a bit much for a nine-year-old to understand. As he begins to learn about sexuality and reproduction, you can introduce the idea that KS may make it necessary for him to father a child in another way, using assisted reproduction or adoption. Emphasize that adults with KS are perfectly capable of having sex with their partners, but that many are unable to produce sperm past early adulthood. This will allow you to begin the conversation about sperm preservation at the right time.

Because sperm samples are obtained by having the teen or young adult produce a semen specimen by masturbation, the procedure will have to be discussed. Although there are few data and little guidance regarding the psychological and developmental impact of sexual experiences of pre- or early teens, questions and advice may be most appropriately handled by a physician (Pediatrician or Pediatric Endocrinologist or Urologist) with whom the boy is comfortable.

Parents of teens will also have to emphasize that while a man with 47,XXY, will have a greatly reduced sperm count, all men with KS need to practice safe sex, and to use condoms unless they are in committed monogamous relationships and they are certain of the health status of their partners.

An additional issue of which parents of teens with KS and health providers should be aware is that there are some adults with KS who do not feel that they are fully male, but have developed as intersex persons. Some adults with KS, although a small minority, prefer to live as females. The significance of this issue was raised in the survey, and it is discussed in more detail on pages 82 to 85 of this guide.

Another issue that many adolescents with KS confront is gynecomastia. Many adolescent boys, regardless of genetic signature, will develop gynecomastia during puberty. Breast tissue is sensitive to both estrogens and androgens (testosterone inhibits breast growth). At the beginning of puberty, the fraction of testosterone converted to estrogen is high enough to stimulate breast growth. Rising testosterone levels reduce the amount of testosterone converted to estrogen and directly inhibit breast growth. Thus, as testosterone levels rise, any breast growth present goes away in most boys and in many with KS. For about 30 percent of males with KS, however, breast development remains and may accelerate, causing discomfort and psychological distress. For KS boys who require testosterone treatment, the high levels inhibit estrogen production and breast growth. Some physicians have had success in treating adolescents with an aromatase inhibitor to reduce the conversion of testosterone to estradiol, and this may lessen gynecomastia.

A physician can help the family to determine if puberty has concluded and remaining gynecomastia is unlikely to resolve on its own. If this is the case, and the boy is distressed about the breast tissue, or if it is painful, obtain a referral to a plastic surgeon with has specialization in correcting gynecomastia and sculpting the male chest. Many insurance companies deny coverage, believing that this is merely cosmetic. Removal of the breast tissue, however, can help to reduce the elevated risk of breast cancer in males with KS as well as reducing discomfort, and it is critical to the mental health of a young man who is devastated by having breasts that he feels he should not have. If your insurer will not pay for the surgery, find a surgeon who will provide a payment plan.

There is far more to adolescence for a teenager with KS than puberty and hormones, although most parents of teens are not really sure of this! The teen will be making choices in friends and activities, and he will be considering his life after high school and trying to take appropriate courses that will lead to his post-secondary goals. There is no question that the teen years are trying ones for most families, and for the teen with KS, they can be truly challenging. By helping him through puberty medically, parents can at least minimize the traumatic effects of incomplete puberty, low testosterone levels, and gynecomastia.

For parents, there are some important goals for the teen years. Continuing to emphasize good health practices is important, especially a good diet that provides adequate calcium and vitamin D to help with the bone mineralization that will help prevent osteoporosis later in life. It is difficult to limit junk food in a teen's diet, but KS can make some teens prone to weight gain, particularly in the abdomen. Parents can try, even though they may not be successful.

It is equally important to continue to help the teen find physical activity and sports that he likes, and to help him build regular exercise into his life. For some teens, individual sports rather than team sports may be more comfortable. Weight-bearing strength training which builds bone density, including upper body work, will always be a necessary part of his life, and parents should reward their teen for continuing to pursue this. Exercise can be as simple as walking, or as complex as hockey or fencing.

Many of the students who do well academically in grade school and early junior high school may find the greater demands of college prep work and the academic preparation for standardized testing for graduation a challenge. Because KS can affect the speed of information recall and processing, bright students can develop difficulty with test-taking. Students with KS may also experience difficulty as high school coursework increasingly calls for written analysis. They may find verbal expression to be difficult, and the process of both developing an essay and writing it down by hand almost impossible. For students who may not have needed any special education services to do the more elementary and basic academic work of earlier years, parents may now need to ask for academic accommodations, such as extra time on tests, or the use of a laptop computer in the classroom for note-taking.

The survey's open-ended questions about educational programs provided many reports of school personnel who had difficulty in understanding the learning difficulties of students with KS. Parents report that many schools termed the boys "lazy" and "underachieving" largely because they have IQs in the normal range, and yet did poorly on academic work. This problem is common to the other SCA conditions, Trisomy X and 47,XYY.

Concrete educational recommendations are included in a later chapter to help support the student in graduating from high school and transitioning successfully to college or to work. Although more than 85 percent of students with KS graduate from high school, there are those who drop out. In North America, the high school dropout can look forward to a life where he has difficulty getting hired, earns less than his peers who graduated, and is more likely to be among the long-term unemployed. Parents of boys with KS who are at risk of not getting a high school diploma may need to take extraordinary measures to make certain that they are able to graduate successfully. Sometimes this means enrolling them in an alternative high school, home-schooling them using online curricula, or helping them to complete a GED.

The transition from high school to adulthood is so important for young persons with extra X and Y chromosomes that it is covered separately in this guide as a chapter. Parents need to do their best to help develop a plan with the school team so that their son graduates from high school and that there are clear plans for post-secondary college, vocational training or work for after graduation. For students with a clear direction and plans for college, or a job lined up after graduating, parents do not need to be concerned. But many high school students with KS have less maturity than their peers, and they may not be at all ready to launch into independent adulthood at the age of 18 or 19. Throughout high school, parents need to remind themselves that while their student may have the same chronological age as his peers, he may be psychologically one or more years behind.

One of the frequent observations of adults with KS, their parents, and the professionals who have performed longitudinal studies is that KS is not itself a developmental disability, but it can be associated with developmental disability and delay. By the age of thirty, however, the majority of adults with KS have "caught up" and managed to establish themselves in jobs and relationships. This seems to happen five to ten years behind "schedule" during adulthood for a significant number of adults with KS. For parents, siblings, partners and professionals who love and work with these men, this is important to remember. It is one good reason not to push them out of high school before they are ready, or demand that they go away to a four year college when they really are only ready to commute to a community college and attend part-time.

This section is written in part to address the requests for information on functioning in adulthood from the parents of adult sons with XXY as well as from the more than 140 adults with mosaic and non-mosaic XXY who responded to the recent survey. It is helpful to review the characteristics of this group of adults with XXY. The average age was 47; seventy-four percent had been diagnosed after age 18. The most frequent reasons for undergoing genetic testing for these individuals were: small testes, 37%; infertility, 26%; and learning, behavior, or psychological problems, 23%. Sixty percent had received special education services in school, with reading services being most common. When asked about bullying, 47% told me that they had been subject to frequent and severe bullying, and 42% had been subject to occasional bullying. Ninety percent had graduated from high school, with nearly half receiving A's and B's in their last academic experience. Seventy-five percent were employed or were now retired, at a range of occupations from professional to skilled trades to unskilled and service employment. Another 25% reported that they had received public disability payments.

I paid careful attention to the adults' answers to open-ended questions. Most were relieved to have finally had a diagnosis to explain puzzling depression and anxiety, and their concerns over bodies that did not develop in the typically masculine manner. They also expressed frustration that so few physicians were familiar with this relatively common genetic condition. The unfamiliarity had delayed diagnosis for a substantial number of them.

The adults also were concerned that much of the knowledge about KS through the lifespan is about children and young adults; there seems to be little knowledge of how KS affects adults who are middle-aged or older. It should be noted that this group of adults represents those in the adult population who can express themselves well verbally. They also are adults who speak English and in some way are associated with support groups. There was significant representation from adults outside of the United States and Canada, including Australia, the United Kingdom, the Netherlands and Scandinavian countries, Japan and a number of other countries.

In contrast to self-reports from the adults, the responses of parents of adults with KS tended not to paint such an optimistic picture of adults who had successfully overcome challenges. Parents reported a higher percentage of adult sons who were receiving disability payments as well as a higher rate of unemployment. Parents were more worried about the lives of their sons, but this may reflect the fact that our respondents were parents who are still fairly involved in their sons' lives, and perhaps have younger sons who still need their assistance, or they have more severely impacted sons who are less able to function independently.

In general, men with KS appear to be satisfied with their lives but report that in terms of career satisfaction and in life relationships, KS has had a rather significant impact. Even if learning disabilities that the men suffered were not severe enough to require special education accommodations or services, there is generally an undertone in responses that academic success for this group of adults requires targeted hard work, including extra time and effort in studying in order to do as well as classmates. Many of those who did college level work noted that they had to overcome difficulties in verbal memory, in speed of verbal recall and processing, and in attention span, in order to perform satisfactorily.

A number of men noted with pride that while it had taken extra years to gain credentials, either a college degree or other vocational experience and training, they had been increasingly motivated to succeed as they became older and more mature. This seems to reflect the experience reported in a 1987 article authored by J. Nielsen and B. Pelsen of Denmark, regarding a follow-up study of 34 Klinefelter males twenty years after the group had first been studied. It should also be noted that in many cases, both the parents of adults and the adults themselves describe lives that had finally "come together" after significant career and personal challenges in early adulthood.

Because of the wide variation in range of functioning as adults, it is impossible to generalize about career success and achievement of overall independence in terms of ability to be self-supporting. The majority of adults with KS, approximately 80 percent, are self-supporting even if settling into a career was somewhat delayed from what they and their parents, in many cases, considered the norm. Given the challenges, academic, social and emotional, that many of these adults have confronted growing up, the fact that such a significant majority has achieved success is a tribute to the resilience and adaptive strength of this population. In many cases, individuals and families have cited acceptance of ones differences as key to "getting on with adult life."

Among the differences cited with which the adults have had to reconcile have been learning disabilities despite normal intelligence, lack of confidence throughout childhood and adolescence, and a sense of insecurity about the "masculinity" of both their bodies and personalities. For some, reconciliation was eased by receiving a diagnosis. For others, the diagnosis was clear, but acceptance required further maturity as well as a significant event, such as meeting the right partner, or discovering a career talent. For the adult with KS, his family and friends, there is a need to exercise patience about his progress toward maturity. Independence may take a longer path than for the typical adult.

A second area of concern is that many adults with KS tell me that they do not feel as though their personalities are consistent with what may be seen as the typical "male": assertive, confident, athletic, and dominant. They feel that they are more sensitive than typically is the case for males. Their confidence has been undermined by awkwardness, both physical and social, as well as difficulties with self-expression. In addition, their strengths are not in either verbal or physical dominance but rather are demonstrated in quieter ways, through interpersonal relationships or by being capable technicians, such as engineers, programmers, carpenters, artists and technical writers. This is where it is important for families to support their adolescents and young adults. Many cited school and workplace bullying as quite painful experiences, with the bullying directed at them, they thought, because of their quiet, sometimes shy, personalities. More painful than the bullying, however, for a limited number, was lack of acceptance by parents, particularly fathers. The extent to which families and persons close to the adult with KS can support him and let him know that he is valued will help him to maximize his progress toward independence, even if his adolescence was somewhat marred by learning and social challenges.

A final recommendation for maximizing functioning as an adult is to obtain high quality medical care to address endocrine and other concerns that are associated with KS. This is a tall order, given that only a small number of dedicated physicians and other health care professionals have developed practices that include specialization in KS and SCA. Because of the small number of these clinicians, it may require the expense and effort of traveling some distance to a university-based consultant for recommendations that can be followed at home by the local physician.

There have been a number of recent breakthroughs in the management and treatment of adolescents and adults with KS. This includes better data regarding determining when and if testosterone therapy is necessary, and certainly better methods of testosterone administration, such as gels, pellets, and underarm applicators. In some cases, additional medications can help to offset the hormonal aberrations result in gynecomastia. Physicians who are current on the latest research know that adults with KS are not necessarily infertile. Some young adolescents have sperm that can be cryopreserved for later use in assisted reproduction. Young adults may also be able to become biological fathers using a variety of techniques. Physicians who have updated knowledge about KS will be aware of conditions that can be associated with KS, such as depression or Type 2 diabetes, and can provide guidance and referrals to address these concerns.

I am an optimist, and I believe that I am seeing what now looks like a slowly growing but accelerating awareness of KS as a highly variable genetic phenotype, one that deserves the attention of researchers, and of professionals in the medical and educational fields. The number of children and adults with the condition is large, even with only 30 percent diagnosed during their lifetimes. Proper awareness by physicians, psychologists and educators of the constellation of symptoms that should cause suspicion about a possible diagnosis may prompt more testing, and earlier and more complete diagnosis.

In the meantime, as a community, we depend on each other for self-education, and to a certain extent, our community will need to take the lead in educating professionals about KS and how to work effectively with this population. I am hopeful that there will be an increasing number of continuing education programs for professionals, such as genetic counselors and family physicians, so that the outdated and inaccurate materials that emphasize criminality and intellectual disability can be replaced by useful information about effective therapies and reduction of risk factors.

I am a bit hesitant to discuss the possible **medical complications** of a genetic condition like KS, for fear of frightening parents as well as adolescents and adults who have recently been diagnosed. This discussion is done with the goal of educating adults and families about health care issues for which they should have a reasoned awareness. That way, they can be on the alert and can educate their own health care providers about screening needs. Individuals and families should be reassured, however, that while there is a slight reduction, less than 2 years on average, in life expectancy in adults with KS, excellent medical care and lifestyle changes, such as weight loss and stopping smoking, can help to minimize the risks of medical conditions associated with KS.

When I surveyed adults about educational needs, the most frequently requested information was on health care implications of KS, particularly in middle age and in the senior years. Parents also commented frequently on the need for guidance about medical and psychiatric issues. Please use this information to help inform health care; don't use it to over-worry about possible health problems. All of us have genetic risk, but most of us do not know what those risks are. In the case of KS, we have some knowledge of possible health care risks and therefore we have the opportunity to make lifestyle and other changes to prevent or minimize future health care problems.

> *I try to find professionals who have at least a basic understanding of KS. If they do not, I educate them. I have found over the years that when you meet doctors and you start to let them know about KS, they will express their desire to want to help physically before saying anything. Taking a step backwards toward*

the door is a good sign that they are not going to want to learn enough to be helpful.

Most doctors I have seen know a few things about XXY, such as what you can read online. I have found it necessary to seek out specialists such as endocrinologists and psycho-pharmacologists who have special training with regard to KS to oversee treatment of the many associated conditions that I seem to have: anxiety, depression, osteoporosis, high cholesterol, etc.

I am concerned that I may have difficulty supporting my wife in the future because of my failing health. I am retired at age 60 because of physical problems that could probably have been avoided had I been treated earlier by more knowledgeable doctors.

Risk in KS appears to result from both hypogonadism, from lower testosterone levels throughout the lifespan, as well as from causes determined at the molecular level because of extra chromosomal material, the "double-dosing" from genes that are not inactivated on the X chromosome. Although it seems fairly clear that osteoporosis, for instance, stems from lowered testosterone levels throughout the lifespan, other possible complications, such as an increased rate of Type 2 diabetes, do not have a clear cause.

The major medical conditions that can affect men with KS disproportionately appear to be osteopenia and osteoporosis; diabetes; elevated cholesterol and lipid levels; autoimmune disorders including lupus; venous ulcers, deep vein thrombosis (blood clots), and peripheral vascular disease; and certain cancers, including breast and lung cancer, and those involving mediastinal (such as lymphoma) and germ cell (testicular) tumors. Dental problems are also well-documented, and in our survey, were reported by over 60 percent of men. In addition, depression and anxiety are also reported by over 60 percent of respondents.

Osteoporosis and osteopenia affect over one-third of all adults. Osteoporosis is a bone condition leading to bone fragility and easy fracture that is defined as a bone mineral density of less than 2.5

standard deviations below the peak bone mass average of healthy, young adults. Osteopenia is a precursor to osteoporosis, and is defined as having a bone density of from 1 to 2.5 standard deviations below the mean for healthy young adults. In older adults, these conditions can lead to hip fracture and to compression fractures of the spine, both of which can contribute substantially to disability and to mortality. Low bone density in boys and adults with KS can be detected in the teens, and appears to be directly related to low testosterone levels, which interfere with complete bone mineralization. The problem is exacerbated by low muscle tone. This can keep the muscles from providing the stressing of bones during weight-bearing exercise that is necessary to build bone density.

The first line of defense against bone-thinning is appropriate supplementation with testosterone. In addition, boys and adults with KS need to engage in regular weight-bearing exercise in order to maintain bone density, along with a good diet and calcium and vitamin D supplements, if recommended. DEXA scans should be performed to monitor bone density. For those who develop osteoporosis or osteopenia, there are other measures that can be taken. A doctor may recommend biphosphenates (Fosamax, Boniva, Reclast) to rebuild bone, although long-term use of these drugs may cause side effects. There is also good medical data that standing and balancing on a vibrating platform for about five minutes daily can substantially improve bone density. Individuals concerned about bone density should also limit their consumption of all sodas, diet and sugared, to one a day because the phosphorus in sodas appears to impede absorption of calcium by bones.

Both Type 1 diabetes and Type 2 diabetes are more common in men with KS than in unaffected men. Type 1 is an autoimmune disorder where the ability of the pancreas to produce insulin is destroyed. The more common type of diabetes, in the general population and in individuals with KS, is Type 2, where the body becomes resistant to insulin. This can be a side effect of obesity, particularly truncal (abdominal) obesity, which affects many adolescents and men with KS. The fat around the middle seems to be an organ in and of itself, and it contributes to the disorder known as metabolic syndrome, characterized by high cholesterol and lipid levels, hypertension, and insulin resistance.

Men with KS, particularly when they have low testosterone levels, are prone to developing metabolic syndrome. Testosterone can decrease the tendency to this disorder, but lifestyle changes, including regular cardiovascular and weight-bearing exercise, as well as adoption of a low-fat and low-carbohydrate, high-protein diet emphasizing whole grains, fruits and vegetables, are really essential to controlling this.

Diet and exercise frequently are not enough for men with KS to control their cholesterol and blood pressure. They may need to follow a doctor's recommendations to take statins to control lipids, as well as medication to control blood pressure. It should be emphasized that it can be extra-difficult for men with KS to control their weight; it isn't the result of a "character flaw," or of not trying harder. There seem to be metabolic issues that affect men with KS that may not affect the general population. Even those men with normal weight in our survey seem to be at greater risk for high cholesterol and lipid levels.

It bears mentioning that there can be psychological and behavioral barriers to maintaining a good diet and an active lifestyle. Some of the symptoms of KS may interfere with the discipline required to stick with a wellness program. Providing supports to the individual, rather than criticism, is more likely to result in successes.

Autoimmune disorders, such as lupus, rheumatoid arthritis, and certain thyroid problems, are significantly more common in men with KS. There are no preventive measures available, nor is there data that testosterone can minimize the risk of developing these problems. There is speculation that because women are at greater risk than men for developing autoimmune disorders, that either the presence of two X chromosomes or higher estrogen levels may contribute to risk.

We know that venous ulcers and peripheral vascular disease are much more common is KS than in the general population. Deep vein thrombosis (DVT) and pulmonary embolism occur more frequently than in the general population, and can affect quite young men with KS as well as older men. The cause of these problems is not completely understood, but either low androgen levels or the effects of extra chromosomal material may impair the blood's natural ability to reduce clotting. Prevention, beyond maintaining overall general good health, is difficult. For those scheduled to undergo elective surgery, it is worth a discussion with the physician about aspirin or another anti-coagulant therapy as a preventive after surgery. Use of compression stockings after surgery may also be a recommended. If an ulcer appears to be developing on the foot or leg, an individual needs to consult a good wound care specialist immediately.

Many physicians are not familiar with KS and its association as a risk factor for DVT and pulmonary embolism, so it will be up to you to educate them. Teens and adults who have KS who are on airline flights of over an hour should try to get up every hour and walk around in order to minimize risk for DVT caused by inactivity in air travel.

Men with KS actually have a lower risk of ischemic cardiac disease (angina or heart attack caused by narrowed arteries or those blocked by a clot) than men overall; their risk is actually closer to that of women, perhaps due to the protective effect of higher estrogen levels.

Men with KS also have a lower risk of prostate cancer than men without KS, but that is probably only because a number of men with KS remain untreated with testosterone. For men who take supplemental testosterone as well as those who do not, prostate cancer remains a risk, and regular prostate exams should be done as recommended by a doctor. The risk of breast and lung cancer is elevated, and there may be increased risk for germ cell (testicular) and mediastinal tumors including lymphoma. Men with KS need to perform regular breast and testicular self-exams. If they smoke, they should do everything possible to stop, because this contributes to vascular disease, in addition to lung cancer.

Dental problems seem to stem from a high rate of taurodontism, a condition in which the enamel is relatively thin and the interior of the teeth, particularly of molars, is large and pulpy. Cavities become severe more quickly in men with KS and some families state that the enamel itself is less strong, and more prone to decay. We know that men and boys with KS spend lots of money on dentists, and that many adults go to extraordinary lengths to retain their teeth, resorting to root canals and caps to prevent loss, and to implants when teeth are lost to gum disease or tooth decay. In fact, dentists are sometimes the clinicians who are first to suggest to a patient that genetic testing for KS may be appropriate, because dental difficulties are so characteristic of the condition.

Advice to minimize dental problems includes making certain that the level of fluoride, either from drinking water or in supplements, or as a result of topical fluoride treatments, is adequate. Careful and lengthy brushing with an electric toothbrush and regular flossing are also recommended. For a number of respondents, a professional cleaning four times a year, rather than twice, is worth the expense, which is usually about $100. Although tooth sealants are usually limited to children, adults with KS may be able to decrease decay by having their dentist apply them. Boys and adults with KS should make a point of telling the dentist that they have Klinefelter syndrome and that their risk of decay and tooth loss is quite elevated. A partnership with the dentist to preserve natural teeth is important for a person with KS.

Additional medical concerns focus on the risk for psychiatric disorders associated with KS. There does appear to be an increased rate of psychiatric difficulty, ranging from ADHD to anxiety and depression, bipolar disorder, and psychotic disorder, including schizophrenia. In childhood, the most commonly reported difficulty is ADHD followed by various anxiety disorders. Depression of varying severity seems to affect the majority of individuals at some time in their lives. For a small minority, there can be a diagnosis of bipolar disorder or of schizophrenia or other thought disorders.

Although testosterone supplementation appears to reduce symptoms in many boys and men, it is by no means a cure. Some men will struggle with anxiety, depression, and more severe disorders throughout their lives. Adults in our survey described medicating themselves with alcohol or illegal drugs in an attempt to reduce their symptoms, although it appears that substance abuse is no more common in persons with KS than in the general population.

We do not know to what extent the emotional problems of individuals with KS are the result of abnormal hormone levels, of the stress of a lifetime of learning and social disabilities, or of something to do with the extra X chromosome and its impact on brain development and brain functioning. We do know that all individuals with extra X and Y chromosomes are at greater risk of these disorders than the general population, which points to the extra chromosome(s) as contributing to the increased risk. It is important for parents to recognize the risk of emotional problems and to take action should signs develop. This is a very clear case in which emotional disorders are not the "fault" of the parents but rather of the interplay of neurological differences, hormonal disturbances, and environmental problems, such as stress at school caused by learning problems or bullying.

For adults, it is important to recognize that supportive counseling and in some cases, medication, may be necessary to help maintain a satisfying life. In almost all cases, the hormonal disturbances of KS need to be addressed along with emotional symptoms, as they appear to be linked. If you encounter a psychiatrist or psychologist who maintains that there is no link between KS and psychiatric disturbances, then find another clinician. As always, teamwork is required to help the individual with KS manage his symptoms in such a way that they do not derail his life.

Fertility and family building also comprise one of the major concerns of adults with KS. It is often said that the most difficult thing to accept for individuals with KS, particularly teens and adults, is that they are probably infertile and will never be able to father biological children. However, recent advances in knowledge about fertility in the males with KS and advances in assisted reproductive technology render this statement untrue.

We now know that boys will produce viable sperm in their ejaculate through the early and mid-teens that can be harvested and cryo-preserved for later use. We also know that adults can have viable sperm within their testicles that can be retrieved through testicular biopsy under a microscope. This sperm can then be injected into eggs (ova) retrieved from the partner to form embryos which can be implanted in the woman's uterus. This is called ICSI, intracytoplasmic sperm injection. The success rate of ICSI has been shown to equal and sometimes exceed the success rate for standard in vitro fertilizations procedures.

It is no longer necessary to announce to an adolescent or young man who has been diagnosed with KS that he is infertile. It can be presented as having decreased fertility that requires special assistance in order to achieve a pregnancy. The knowledge that most young teens have viable sperm in their ejaculate and that it can be cryo-preserved is fairly recent. Parents of teens can investigate this with any endocrinologist or urologist who normally performs sperm preservation with children who are scheduled to undergo chemotherapy. If this is being considered, it is best to do this as soon as possible after puberty because there is a sudden fall-off in production of sperm, often by age fifteen, in most boys with KS as their testes begin to fail and their LH and FSH levels rise.

In all men with cells that make sperm, high levels of testosterone within the testis are required for these cells to divide and complete the process of sperm production. When testosterone is used to treat low levels by any method, the amount of testosterone inside the testis falls to a level that may be too low for successful sperm production. However, in adult men with KS who have been treated with testosterone, stopping the treatment for a period of time allows successful retrieval of sperm by biopsy. Although cryo-preserved sperm may be viable for twenty years or more, cryopreserved sperm from KS boys have not been studied. The costs of maintaining the frozen sperm were about $2400 for a ten-year period in 2011, but the cost varies widely.

For adults who are anticipating a pregnancy with their partners, the most important thing is to consult a fertility center that has experience working with men with KS and other problems that produce a low sperm count. We will probably begin to hear within this decade about young men who will have their frozen sperm from their teen years thawed and used to fertilize their partners' eggs in petri dishes. Currently, however, most adult men with KS who work with a fertility specialist will have testicular sperm extraction (TESE), following treatment which often requires them to discontinue the use of testosterone and take one or more drugs, such as aromatase inhibitors, that will help their testes function well enough to produce sperm. The partner will have her ovaries stimulated with drugs to produce multiple ova (eggs), and the ova will be retrieved surgically one day, while the man will have TESE the following day. Once sperm are obtained, ICSI (intracytoplasmic sperm injection) will be performed to fertilize the eggs.

Because men with KS tend to produce a higher percentage of sperm that have additional X and Y chromosomes, it may be recommended that couples who undergo ICSI have "pre-implantation diagnosis" of the embryos that result, prior to selecting those to insert in the woman's uterus. This involves removing one cell from an eight-cell embryo, and testing it for the presence of extra chromosomes. If any 47,XXY, or 47,XXX, embryos are detected, they are not implanted.

In one study, the mean age of men with KS involved in TESE and ICSI was age 33. In 54 TESE attempts with 42 patients, 69 percent of patients had sperm retrieved. The mean number of oocytes (eggs) injected was 7.7 of which 4.6 oocytes on average were fertilized. Eighteen pregnancies were achieved, a 46 percent success rate, and 21 babies were born of these pregnancies. It is estimated that the cost of each cycle involving TESE and ICSI costs approximately $25,000, which may or may not be covered by insurance policies. Embryos that are not implanted in the current cycle can be frozen as can sperm not used to fertilize eggs for that cycle, for later attempts, but the success rate for pregnancies is lower with either frozen embryos or with frozen sperm.

Couples have always had the option of using donor sperm, and many couples with KS have achieved parenthood with this option, as have those who have adopted children. Development of the protocols permitting men with KS to father biological children, however, provides an additional option, as does the practice of cryopreservation of sperm in a boy's teenage years.

I developed two open-ended questions for the adults who took the survey to ask them to comment on **sexuality and relationships**. The questions asked whether being 47,XXY, had affected relationships in general, and whether they believed that having 47,XXY, had affected their sexuality or their gender identity. I had always wanted to understand the issue, because this is one of the most controversial in the XXY community. Parents, particularly, want desperately to believe that KS in no way will make their sons more likely to identify as "gay" or as "female." At the same time, a substantial number of adults with KS are quite openly gay, and some live, again openly, as women. My survey did not attempt to measure the proportion, to try to determine if the percentage exceeded the ten percent estimate of homosexuality in the population. I simply wanted to hear from adults who are given anonymity what their opinions were.

The questions were answered by 117 adults with KS. Remember that this population in the survey had an average age of 46, and that they are quite articulate; it may be that a truly scientific sample would look a bit different. A self-identified sample is not scientifically and statistically valid because there is no guarantee that its characteristics (age, education, socioeconomic status, etc.) are representative of the larger population.

Two thirds of the adults stated that having KS had affected the quality of their relationships with other people, largely because of communication difficulties, both verbal and non-verbal. They felt that they tended to be somewhat shy and introverted, and that their insecurity in their "maleness" as younger adolescents and as teens had colored their adult relationships. Some felt that they had held back a bit, because they always felt that they had been somewhat "different."

In terms of sexuality issues, sexual preference, and gender identity, slightly less than two-thirds thought that having KS had had a significant impact on their lives. About forty per cent said that KS had had negligible impact on sexual issues in their lives. Of those who did state that KS was significant in this realm, a number stated that they were gay, but this group was divided about whether they thought that KS had any role in sexual preference. Four persons stated that they lived as women, and that they had preferred to identify as girls even when young. Those living as women resent the common medical advice for KS men to use testosterone, and all four XXYs living as women prefer to use estrogen for health reasons. More common, however, were statements of some gender confusion in adolescence, because of having small genitalia and developing gynecomastia.

> *I would say, being an XXY, that I am more caring and compassionate towards others than many men. I also have a strong need to help others. My wife and I get along fine, and she feels she wouldn't want to have married an XY after experiencing the calmness and caring of an XXY.*
>
> *I don't believe it has had an effect on my sexuality or gender identity. I am a man with all physical signs pointing to it. I do seem more emotional than most other men, but I don't see this as a negative. I see it as a positive attribute.*
>
> *I've always thought of myself as male, but I do exhibit some stereotypical female tendencies.*
>
> *How does one separate ones sexual and gender identity from ones overall identity? I am who I am and since I believe being XXY has profoundly affected who I am it would also profoundly affect my sexuality and gender identity. Since getting T therapy I am more confident in declaring myself male but with caveats. Sexuality-wise I sometimes classify myself with autogynephilia but non-sexually I see myself as male. Gender confusing perhaps?*

Often, the answer focused on questions about sexuality because of having a low sex drive, or having little attraction to women. After diagnosis and treatment with testosterone, some began to feel fully "male," and were able to communicate with their partners much better about their sexuality issues. They began to understand why things might have been so confusing for them in their younger years when they felt "different." In most men who found sexuality easier and more satisfying after diagnosis, they became more attracted to women. In a small minority, they came to terms more easily with either bisexuality or homosexuality.

Another small group contends that sexually and emotionally, they are "intersex." They contend that they are divided between masculine and feminine in their approach not only to sexuality but also in their approach to life, in their relationships with others, and in their preferences for leisure activities. Medically, "intersex" refers to having ambiguous genitalia neither fully masculine nor fully feminine. But this group of adults believes that while they may have male genitalia, their brains are truly "intersex." The purpose of my survey was not to argue semantics; I wished to listen to what adults with these conditions have to say, and a number of adults told me the same thing.

> *I knew I was gay before I knew I was XXY. If anything, being XXY keeps me from stereotypical gay behavior. I will not have sex with "just anyone."*
>
> *I was never very coordinated. I was shy, and I didn't have that rough, tough attitude that a lot of guys have. This I know is from having low testosterone. I am attracted to men, yes, but I am not completely gay... it is hard to explain. I do believe though that having an extra X chromosome thrown in there may have something to do with it. I believe that attraction may be genetic in the end. I can't say definitely that if I didn't have KS I would be any different sexually, as both men with and without KS are gay, bi and straight, but I do believe that it has affected me personally.*

At first, I thought I was born the wrong sex. I felt more like a girl and thought that maybe I should undergo a sex change because I was in love with boys and then men. I was attracted to boys when I was as young as in the fourth grade. Then I discovered the term "gay" and I then decided that I did not need a sex change because if I were gay, I could have a teenage boy when a teenager, and a man when I became an adult. Now I don't care what I am called, but I use the term XYX.

We seem to be seeing in some adults with KS a very real variation in sexuality and in gender identity that may be due to in part to the extra X chromosome itself and in part to variations in hormone levels at various points during the lifespan. The compassionate view has to be that adults who may have been born with these differences or who have developed these differences over their lives, are expressing very real emotions about sexuality and gender identity. It doesn't help for parents, who hope that their children will be spared the angst of this uncertainty, to deny that these questions may exist for many boys and men with KS. If their children are having such questions as they grow up, they should be acknowledged and helped to reconcile with their feelings. Adults with 47,XXY, may become more comfortable with the advocacy organizations if those who have leadership roles in them could feel safe discussing these issues. As with all things surrounding KS and 47,XXY, there is enormous variation in whether individuals have questions about their sexuality or their gender identity. The majority of adults with KS do not, but there is certainly a group for whom these questions continue to be an issue.

Klinefelter Syndrome Variations (48,XXYY; 48,XXXY; and 49,XXXXY)

Approximately 10 percent of boys and men with Klinefelter syndrome have a **variation** (48,XXXY; 48,XXYY; and 49,XXXXY),rather than the typical genetic signature, 47,XXY. These men and boys have either 48 or 49 chromosomes rather than 47 chromosomes. Variants involving four chromosomes instead of the XY pair are sometimes referred to as *tetrasomy XY*, and those involving five chromosomes, as *pentasomy XY*. In general, men and boys who have one of the variants will have more severe learning, behavioral and physical disabilities. It is estimated that each additional X chromosome will reduce the full-scale IQ by about 15 points. There is still a significant range of functioning within each of the variations. Boys with variant signatures of KS are more likely to be diagnosed in childhood because they may have distinctive facial features that lead pediatricians to request genetic testing, as well as more pronounced speech and developmental delays than with 47,XXY.

Adults with variations of KS benefit from support through organizations for persons with learning disabilities and mild intellectual disability. They are often capable of holding part-time jobs, and many can live independently in an apartment with supervision. Because they tend to be passive (and often eager to build relationships at any cost), safeguards should be instituted so that they are not subject to financial scams or other exploitation. Men with variant karyotypes have all of the medical risks of KS, including venous ulcers, osteoporosis, diabetes, male breast cancer and autoimmune disorders. Medical supervision should include regular visits to a primary care doctor who is aware of KS as a risk factor, and screening regularly for possible complications. They should have a supervised nutrition and exercise program focused on reducing the risk of complications from obesity and osteoporosis.

The most common of the variant conditions, **48,XXYY,** is actually considered to be a clinical and genetic condition distinct from Klinefelter syndrome, because of particular physical and psychological characteristics that occur only in XXYY men. The condition, however, shares many of the same phenotypic characteristics, including tall stature, testicular failure, speech delay and learning disability, as both non-variant and variant KS.

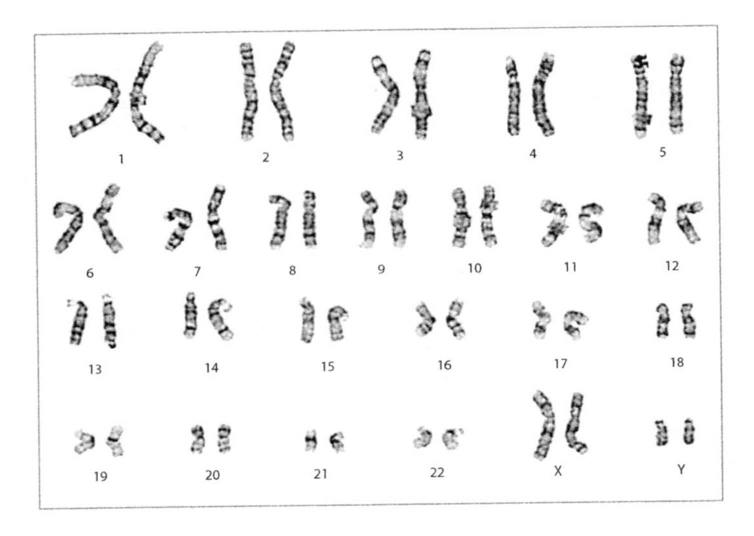

Karyotype of 47,XXYY
[Used with permission of Colorado Genetics]

Although men with XXYY have lower IQ scores than normal for the population, only one-third score in the range of intellectual disability, typically an adult IQ score of less than 70. Learning disabilities, however, tend to be significant in this group, and most often are also accompanied by ADHD, which affects over 70 percent. Autism spectrum disorders have been reported in 28% of children with XXYY.

Men with XXYY are usually tall, and mean height exceeds that for men with 47,XXY. They may have mild facial dysmorphia, including an *epicanthic fold* of the upper eyelid covering the inner corner of the eye; mild *hypertelorism,* or a noticeably greater distance between the eyes than the width of the eye; prominent nasal bridge; and sometimes, unusual ear shapes. Some have quite prominent teeth or severe malocclusion, necessitating extensive orthodontia. In addition, many parents indicated that their boys had abnormally thin enamel and were prone to early and severe dental decay.

Other physical abnormalities are more common in and pronounced in men and boys with XXYY. Almost half of those in our survey had *radio-ulnar synostosis*, or difficulty in straightening out the elbows. *Clinodactyly* (curved little finger) was also more common in XXYY than in 47,XXY. A significant number also suffer from *hypospadius* (urethra located above or below the penis instead of at the end of the penis), *cryptorchidism* (undescended testicle) and *micropenis*. Cardiac problems affect between 15 and 20 percent. A number of boys and men also suffer from respiratory disorders, including asthma and recurrent pneumonia, which may be related to *hypotonia* and difficulty in clearing the lungs, particularly in children. Hand tremors are also more common and more pronounced, particularly as men with XXYY move into their 20s.

> *He is a very compassionate person and he is a pleaser. He never ceases to amaze me in how, even though I didn't think he could achieve something, he manages to do it successfully.*
>
> *My son is caring, a great artist, and a wonderful cook. Tonight he is going to cook a meal for the whole family, and he'll do it himself, and it will taste great.*
>
> *He does not learn by listening, so we worked really hard to get him reading well. He learns well from written and visual materials. He is interested in nature, outdoor active pursuits, and manual work. Although he doesn't have good fine motor control, he has enjoyed metalwork and woodwork, and is gaining skills as a handyman around the house.*

Although there have been reports of boys and men with XXYY being aggressive, this is not a typical characteristic. While generally pleasant and somewhat shy, boys and men with XXYY can have a low frustration tolerance, and can be impulsive. Many also display considerable anxiety. They often want to have their world well-ordered, and they become upset when there are sudden and unexpected changes. They tend to have difficulties in self-regulating their behavior, and can show a great deal of anger, particularly when bullied. Because their cognitive level is in the low-normal/borderline range, boys with XXYY are often mainstreamed in school with special help. They are not usually in "sheltered" settings, and thus come into contact with the all of the typical social stresses of school. Their immaturity, however, may make it difficult for them to navigate the social demands of a typical school or work setting. Frustrated outbursts, however, are far more likely than physical aggression. Mood dysregulation is fairly common, and often requires a combination of medications for control, including anti-depressants, anti-anxiety agents, mood stabilizers, and anti-psychotic medications. Some adolescents and adults suffer from bi-polar depression, although most have less severe mood swings and cyclothymic disorders.

Boys with XXYY can benefit from a program of speech, physical and occupational therapies to improve their communication skills and to allow them to develop more age-appropriate fine and gross motor skills. Their difficulties with sustaining attention may require stimulant or other medication, along with placement in a smaller class setting. A small, well-organized and structured classroom may also help to address their difficulties with anxiety.

Parents who responded to the survey were adamant that bullying of their sons needed to be avoided at all costs, as bullying created enormous anxiety in their sons, leading to school phobia and considerable distress even at home. Even for those without a diagnosis of autism spectrum disorder, the speech therapy and social skills training techniques developed for autistic persons of using social stories and scripting can be very effective for this population. In addition to building their vocabularies, teaching the use of language for social purposes can help them to handle social situations more effectively, without resorting to outbursts.

Some physicians have been reluctant to prescribe testosterone supplementation for adolescents and adults with XXYY, fearing that it will make these males aggressive. Testosterone, however, has a similar impact in XXYY males as in XXY males. The hormone often improves bone density, reduces anxiety and depression, improves stamina, and increases muscle mass. For men with XXYY who are hypogonadal, testosterone is a necessary therapy and, provided that the dosage is appropriate, should not produce aggression.

The majority of men with XXYY qualify for disability income benefits, although half of the men in our survey also worked part-time at a variety of unskilled jobs, such as landscaping, packaging and food service. The concerns of parents of these men is that while their adult sons can be partially independent, and some live on their own in apartments, most will always need some level of supervision and support.

> *My greatest concern is about his ability to live independently of me, whether in a group setting or otherwise. I am always concerned for his safety as he is very innocent and trusting even of strangers.*
>
> *Our son is currently on our health insurance but when we retire, health insurance will be an issue for him. He is currently living at home but is capable of living on his own, but can't afford to. There is a "catch 22" to SSI where our son is able to work but makes too much for SSI (which would give him Medicaid) but too little to afford health insurance.*

While most governments provide a safety net and ongoing services for those with "borderline" developmental disabilities, many have comprehensive services only for those who have clear intellectual disability or who have persistent and severe psychiatric disorders. Many XXYY men do not fit into either of these categories.

The XXYY Project, founded in 1998, provides families with information about effective treatment modalities, helps families to develop IEPs specific to the needs of an XXYY child, and provides other supports to families developing employment and independent living arrangements for their sons. The Project also sponsors an annual symposium for families. Information is available at www.xxyysyndrome.org

48, XXXY, is a true variant of Klinefelter syndrome. As in XXYY, there can be mild facial dysmorphia, including epicanthal eye folds, hypertelorism, pronounced overbite, and slight ear irregularities. Stature may be tall, but is more likely to be in the normal range, although the legs and arms tend to be disproportionately long. Mild intellectual disability is common, with IQ in the range of 40 to 60. Most have significant speech delay as toddlers and well as delayed motor development. Their coordination, fine motor skills, and verbal abilities remain poor throughout life. These males often have underdeveloped genitalia and are hypogonadal, requiring testosterone supplementation.

Boys and men with XXXY tend to be shy and quiet. Speech therapy should be directed at helping them to improve their vocabularies and their ability to interact socially. Using social stories and teaching scripted language appropriate to the situation is also an effective means of helping them interact socially. There are no specific pronounced behavioral difficulties, although attention problems have been noted along with a tendency to depression. Boys tend to be immature for chronological age, and the immaturity extends into adulthood.

I am a sibling and guardian for my brother. Our parents are now deceased, but I remember my mother stating that after she got the MR diagnosis, the recommendation was that my brother be placed in an institution, as it was not likely that he would ever walk or talk. (Strangely, the diagnosis of KS did not happen until years later.) Instead, my mother began a nursery school for handicapped children, and my brother certainly learned to walk and talks quite a bit! He does have osteoporosis now, but as a child did well running in Special Olympics. He lives in a small home setting nearby and comes to stay with my husband and me every weekend.

Being rais Mentally Retarded, I learn nothing. Then I found out I was a rare XXXY. Using the computer I now hear from other XXXY and am not alone now. I am not as dumb as parents thout. Too bad this computer wasn't around when I was in Specal Ed.

The variant form of KS with the most severe symptoms and presentation is **49,XXXXY.** Many of these children are diagnosed in infancy because they present with facial dysmorphic features including hypertelorism, epicanthic eye folds, a broad nose, and low-set and malformed ears. Sometimes there is cleft palate. The neck can be short and broad. They can have *microcephalia* (small head and abnormally small brain). Cardiac defects are found in 15–20 percent. Many have short stature. They also may have a variety of skeletal malformations including radioulnar synostosis and hyperextensible joints. Genitals are almost always underdeveloped and some present with ambiguous genitalia.

Children with 49,XXXXY, may be born small and may be hypotonic. They usually have significantly delayed language and motor skill development. They have IQs ranging from 20 to 60 but most are in the range of moderate intellectual disability. Receptive language is usually greater than expressive language. Some children and adults never develop functional speech and may rely on augmentative communication devices such as chat boards.

I recommend sign language as soon as possible. I recommend that parents learn as much as possible about the child's diagnosis and about dyspraxia and apraxia. The parents need to be strong advocates for their child with doctors, therapists, and school personnel. You must get to know as much as possible about his strengths and weaknesses to do this. Contact other families to learn more. This has helped us tremendously.

These children and adults are usually somewhat quiet and shy although generally pleasant. They can become irritable, however, and may have temper tantrums. They have a low frustration tolerance and similar to persons with autism, have difficulty when there are deviations from routine. Some of these individuals also have a diagnosis of mild autism (often Pervasive Developmental Disorder) because their behaviors and sensory processing difficulties produce similar symptoms, including flapping and other stereotypic movements. Some prefer repetitive activities and find them soothing.

I most admire his determination, his sense of humor and his willingness to share. He does everything that his older brother does. He has an awesome memory and even reminds me of things that I forget.

Our son works in a sheltered workshop and is quite happy being with his friends.

He loves music and swimming, and he is very good with using computers and games. He has a very pleasant and friendly character. A real joy to have in the household.

Adolescents and adults with 49,XXXXY, may benefit from testosterone, although it is not always helpful and may lead to inappropriate sexual behavior. It should be prescribed under the supervision of an experienced endocrinologist and the dosage adjusted as necessary. These adults generally will need supervision in a residential setting. They may require behavior plans to minimize tantrums and occasionally psychotropic medication to help manage their behavior. Some are able to work in well-structured and supervised job placements. Parents of children and young adults with 49,XXXXY, compare their functioning level with that of individuals with Down syndrome. There is a significant range of functioning, from those who are able to hold jobs and walk to and from work independently, to those who require constant supervision.

Parents of children and adults with 49,XXXXY, share several list-serves and online sites including www.xxxxysyndrome.com.

47,XYY, Syndrome

Sometimes mistakenly thought to be a variation of Klinefelter syndrome, 47,XYY, is a distinct condition that only rarely involves the hypogonadism and infertility that KS produces. The condition is occasionally called Jacobs syndrome, but that term is not in wide use. It is believed to occur in 1 in 1,000 male births, and causes few detectable physical signs in either newborns or in older children and adults beyond tall stature. The extra Y chromosome is always contributed by the father, and can occur either during spermatogenesis, when the chromosomes in the dividing cells fail to separate properly, or it can occur after fertilization. The risk of XYY does not increase with advancing paternal age. Mosaic XYY can occur, with the most common mosaicism being 46,XY/47,XYY. XYY boys and men can be completely symptom-free, but they can also have significant language impairment and developmental and emotional difficulties.

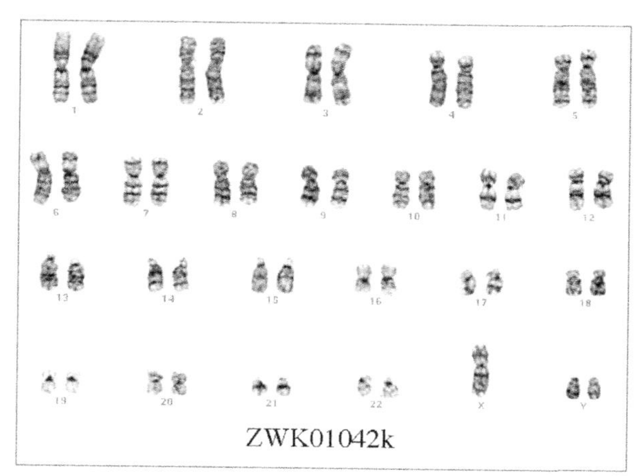

Karyotype of 47,XYY
[Used with permission of the Wisconsin State Laboratory of Hygiene, Board of Regents of the University of Wisconsin System]

Diagnosis is usually made because of language delay, or developmental or emotional difficulties, although some boys are diagnosed prenatally. It is estimated that the percentage of men with 47,XYY, who are diagnosed over a lifetime is about 12 percent, considerably less than for KS, which is about 30 percent. This is because XYY rarely affects either puberty or fertility. Boys with XYY generally go through puberty normally, although there are a small number reported who do not and require supplemental testosterone. As is the case with most of the SCA conditions, there is neither dysmorphia nor any other clear physical sign that would lead pediatricians or other professionals to suspect a genetic disorder.

> *My son's preschool screened him at 2½. He was in early intervention before I knew about the XYY, due to his speech problems and the need for occupational and physical therapy to address his motor skill delay and hypotonia. Initially, he was classified as Speech Impaired. At age 5, when we got the XYY diagnosis, his classification changed to Other Health Impaired (OHI).*
>
> *The broad range of abilities of kids with SCA should be emphasized. Each child needs to be treated as an individual. We had been warned about behavior problems with XYY boys, but this is just not true for our son. He is sweet and polite and well-liked by others in his class. He almost never gets in trouble at school, and if he does, it is for something like forgetting homework, not for bad behavior.*
>
> *He is polite, thoughtful and compassionate. In school, he excels at math, science and reading. He's popular with students and teachers. As a mother, I like his sensitivity and caution.*

If XYY does lead to symptoms, there is considerable overlap with symptoms that characterize KS, including speech delay, hypotonia and difficulty with motor skill development, attention problems, and learning disabilities. There are, however, subtle and important differences. We do not know as much about boys with XYY as boys with

KS because some of the more well-known longitudinal studies did not include enough cases of XYY to form any conclusions. A recent study by Dr. Judith Ross and others, however, did detailed cognitive and motor evaluations on these boys and provides a considerable amount of data, as well as comparisons between boys with XXY and boys with XYY.

Overall, full scale IQ does not appear to be significantly diminished for boys with XYY, compared with siblings, but verbal IQ tends to be lower than performance IQ. Boys with XYY tend to have delayed speech development, and continue to have difficulties with word retrieval, speed of language processing, verbal memory, and both oral and written expressive language. Receptive language is usually better than expressive language, but the ability to interpret what is being conveyed remains a problem, because the boys often have difficulty understanding, for instance, figurative or metaphorical language, as well as complex sentence structures. Children with XYY may also have attention-related problems in that they can be easily distracted and may have difficulty switching their attention from one thing to another.

Coordination problems can exist and often affect handwriting. Some babies and children with XYY are affected by hypotonia which slows their development of sitting, crawling and walking skills. Of individuals in our survey, hypotonia and motor skill deficits were noted as a problem for two-thirds of individuals. Tremors and tics were noted in 25 percent, and seizures in 12 percent. ADHD affected 53 percent, and anxiety, 45 percent. As with other SCA conditions, severe tooth decay was noted frequently as a problem. SCA appears to affect the composition of the enamel, making it less resistant to decay.

When two groups of boys, one with KS (47,XXY) and the other with 47,XYY, were compared, the boys with XYY tended to have more severe and pervasive language impairment than the boys with KS. Boys with XYY also performed less well at reading. XYY boys, in contrast to those with KS, had less impairment in their motor functioning on measures of strength, speed and coordination. In general, however, the measures that parents and schools would take to assist young children and school age boys with XYY in developing appropriate motor, speech and social skills are very similar to those recommended for parents of boys with KS and girls with Trisomy X. This involves creating significant opportunity to develop gross and fine motor skills in a non-competitive setting. Reading to children every day helps them to develop vocabulary and to learn about language in a very effective way. Limiting the use of television and DVDs as entertainment and substituting instead activities like puzzle time, music, cooking, and physical exercise will help the boy to develop skills that can help him to compensate for learning disabilities and social skill deficits.

It may be useful for parents of boys with 47,XYY, to read the previous section on 47,XXY, on infancy, early childhood and school age years, disregarding the sections on difficulties in going through puberty and needing hormone treatment. The early developmental, educational and social issues that can impact boys with XYY and boys with XXY can be quite similar, and require very similar parental approaches. Issues regarding puberty rarely affect boys with XYY, but if they do, and the boy requires testosterone supplementation, the section on XXY, puberty, and testosterone treatment, will provide some background for the boy and his parents.

It is important for a child with mild disabilities to have safe opportunities for socialization where he will not be bullied or treated badly because of his differences. He should be able to count on his family members to be supportive and accepting. If necessary, find other appropriate groups associated with his school, youth groups and local disabilities organizations, as well as religious organizations, so that you and he can do activities in a relaxed atmosphere. Social skills training can help the boy who has difficulty expressing himself effectively, and who has difficulty in reading the social cues of other children.

Early intervention is seen as critical for these children, many of whom have significant language delay. For those with other behavioral or physical concerns, some parents reported that they had difficulty in obtaining occupational or physical therapy because these delays were more subtle and less pronounced than the speech problems. Professionals generally have a very limited understanding of the implications of a diagnosis of XYY for developmental problems, so that even when a prenatal diagnosis or diagnosis in early childhood exists, it may not help with qualifying for services, unless the parent takes measures to educate the professionals about the range of delays that XYY can produce.

Of boys with XYY referred for developmental evaluation at one clinic, nearly 30 percent met the criteria for autism spectrum disorder, usually a milder autism presentation such as PDD-NOS (Pervasive Developmental Disorder-Not Otherwise Specified). There are occasional reports of boys with XYY who never develop functional language although this is rare. Of the 62 XYY cases in our survey, 20 were reported to have an autism spectrum disorder, and several were characterized as "severe." It has only been in recent years that a link between autism and XYY or any of the other sex chromosome aneuploidy conditions has been made, but these cases are usually milder forms of autism spectrum disorders, rather than classical autism.

It is important for parents of infants and young children with the diagnosis of 47,XYY, to tell the pediatrician of the risk for development of autism spectrum disorder, and to make certain that their child has regular screening for meeting developmental milestones. If a boy with XYY begins to show signs of not meeting those milestones on time, aggressive action to obtain early intervention services is the best way to minimize the impact of the condition.

> *Social stories, visual aids such as calendars and schedules, an assistive communication device, behavior modeling and a consistent behavior program have all been very helpful. The structure of ABA is very good for teaching academics.*

Applied Behavior Analysis (ABA) therapy is a well-researched methodology for working with children and adults with autism and other developmental disabilities. Early intervention using ABA techniques can help to foster language and appropriate social behavior in children diagnosed with autism spectrum disorders. Many of the parents of children with XYY as well as autism have spoken highly of the use of ABA in helping their children to develop more normally.

School age concerns continue to center on language-based learning difficulties, and now expand to involve reading, spelling, and writing difficulties. Parents often identify social skill deficits in their children that are associated with communication difficulties and immature behavior compared with peers. Parents also note that as school work and directions given by teachers become more complex, their boys have more difficulty understanding all elements of the instructions, and have difficulty with being able to complete assignments appropriately. Elementary school is also the point at which ADHD and impulsivity can become a problem, particularly if the boy is disruptive in class.

> *Our son was finally put in a fully self-contained educational setting. His 7th grade teacher was the first to suggest chromosome testing, and our son was then diagnosed at age 13. The school system has been proactive in learning more about his condition and developing effective ways to teach him.*
>
> *My son is happy and self-confident. He is very social and funny and engaging. He will shut down in school if he does not understand a subject, but if someone is willing to sit with him and give him individual attention, he can focus, understand and master it.*

Children with XYY are usually of normal or somewhat increased height in infancy and as young children. This increase in height usually accelerates between ages 6 and 9, and then at puberty, many become extraordinarily tall, with most having a height that exceeds the 75th percentile. This can be a disadvantage for boys who may have learning disabilities and social immaturity, because their height and appearance make them look older than their chronological age. At the same time, their "emotional" ages can be lower than their chronological ages. This may need to be pointed out explicitly to the school so that expectations for their behavior and academic performance are more realistic.

It should be noted that many boys with XYY really have few academic or behavioral concerns, especially in elementary school years. Nearly 30 percent require no special education services. Many go on to stable work or to four-year colleges after high school. However, 30 percent in our sample also carry a diagnosis of autism spectrum disorder, even though it is usually the mild presentation, and a substantial number of boys are receiving treatment for ADHD and are more likely to have impulsivity and behavioral problems.

> *I worry about my son's lack of social skills and whether he will be able to control his moods and his responses to situations so that he can get and keep a job, and so that he can find and keep a life partner. I have already created a mental picture of having him live at home and hold some type of less rigorous job while contributing to the household. That could work.*

At this point, so little research has been done on XYY that we have only the most general of ideas as to why there can be so much variation in expression of this syndrome. Unlike sex chromosome aneuploid conditions involving one or more extra X chromosomes, where much of the extra chromosomal material is inactivated, the extra Y chromosome remains completely activated. We know, then, that phenotypic characteristics are caused by double-dosing of genes on the Y chromosome. We do not know why some individuals are so much more severely affected than others.

A very small number of boys and men with XYY do not make enough testosterone to go through puberty normally, or become hypogonadal as adults. They require testosterone supplementation. We also do not know why this small group is so affected.

Approximately 40 percent of teenage boys with XYY have severe cases of acne, with significant infection and risk of scarring. Parents need to be aware of this risk, and have their son referred to a dermatologist who can treat the condition with effective measures if acne presents as a problem.

Men with XYY usually have normal fertility. The risk for contributing sperm with an extra chromosome is low, because the extra chromosome is usually eliminated in spermatogenesis. Men who are considering pregnancy with their partners, however, may want to have a genetic consultation regarding any risks of aneuploidy in their offspring. Men with XYY also are not known to have any substantial medical risks, although there does appear to be some additional psychiatric risk, primarily for anxiety, depression and substance abuse. It is also possible that adults with XYY are at a somewhat increased risk of psychotic disorders, including schizophrenia and bipolar disorder.

Our sample of XYY cases included 46 percent who had been diagnosed prenatally. We had access to a number of parents who related what they were told by genetic counselors and obstetricians prior to the child's birth. It was generally said that the child would be tall, and might have some learning disabilities. Many were told that if one were going to have a sex chromosome disorder, XYY is the one with the fewest potential problems. Some professionals cited the studies that predicted "criminal behavior" and counseled in favor of termination of the pregnancy, while others provided background that the studies leading to conclusions about increased risk of criminal behavior were highly flawed and should be disregarded. A number of parents were told that they should never, ever reveal the diagnosis because of the link of XYY with criminal tendencies. Few were counseled regarding the extent of developmental delay that does affect some boys, nor that the child might be at risk of psychiatric disorders, including anxiety and depression.

There are relatively few studies of children with XYY, and almost none that follow these children into adulthood. One that did follow boys into early adulthood was done specifically to answer the question of whether boys with KS and boys with XYY were more likely to engage in criminal behavior than their peers. The study subjects were "unselected" individuals identified through infant screening in Scotland, so that there would be no ascertainment bias using data from individuals who already had been shown to have developmental or behavioral problems. The study found that boys with XYY, largely those with lowered IQ, were somewhat more likely to engage in antisocial behavior than either typically developing peers or boys with KS. Antisocial behavior included impulsive property crimes, such as vandalism, and minor theft, not violent crimes such as robbery or assault. We do know that children with XYY are more likely than their peers to be affected by ADHD and to suffer from low esteem associated with learning difficulties and social skill deficits. These conditions with can prompt "acting out" in adolescents and young adults but they are in no way associated with serious and violent criminal behavior. In the study, the only subject who had been convicted of a violent crime, one involving use of a handgun, was an XY control. None of the XYY or XXY men had been charged with anything other than petty theft, vandalism including graffiti, public drunkenness, and other relatively minor offenses.

Our study showed an enormous range of adult ability and functioning level. Adult occupations range from accountant, university administrator, engineer, truck driver and groundskeeper, to those with severe autism who are completely disabled. Two-thirds graduated from high school. Thirty-seven percent of XYY adults qualify for government disability benefits. Only three adults with XYY answered the survey themselves, so it is impossible to form any conclusions from such a small group.

There are some very rare variations on XYY, including 48,XYYY; 49,XXYYY; and 49,XYYYY. The number of reported cases of these variations is too small to draw conclusions, but each extra Y chromosome is associated with increasing cognitive and physical disability. (XXYY is described previously as a separate clinical and genetic syndrome, but some argue that it is more similar to severely impacted males with XYY than to men with XXY.)

For the majority of individuals with XYY, there will probably be academic, social, emotional or vocational concerns, of varying intensity. Even for those boys who get through high school with relatively little difficulty, transition to adulthood can be a time of additional stresses as the young man is forced to "get it all together" in order to achieve independence. The chapters about psychosocial issues, education and transition to adulthood that follow the descriptions of the sex chromosome aneuploid groups provide more specific recommendations for meeting these challenges.

Trisomy X, Tetrasomy X and Pentasomy X

The sex chromosome aneuploid conditions affecting girls and women are Trisomy X, Tetrasomy X and Pentasomy X. Trisomy X, or 47,XXX, is the most common. Its variations are 48,XXXX (Tetrasomy X), and 49,XXXXX (Pentasomy X). These are analogous to Klinefelter syndrome, 47,XXY, and its 48- and 49- chromosome variations, in which each extra X is associated with increasing cognitive and physical disability.

Trisomy X is believed to occur in 1 in 1,000 female births. As in Klinefelter syndrome, the rate of occurrence increases with maternal age. About ninety percent of Trisomy X cases are non-mosaic. Mosaicism occurs in 10 percent, generally 46,XX/47,XXX, but occasionally, 45,X/47,XXX, providing a Turner syndrome cell line, cells having a 45,X, genetic signature. Other mosaicism also occurs, such as 47,XXX/48,XXXX, but it is much less common.

Trisomy X is characterized by the significant range in functioning that marks non-variant Klinefelter syndrome and XYY. Symptoms can be completely absent, they can be mild and limited to motor skill and learning difficulties, or they can be global in nature, and partially disabling. At this time, only an estimated 10 percent of females with Trisomy X are diagnosed in their lifetimes. Prenatal diagnosis may detect 10 percent of the total diagnosed. The remaining cases are diagnosed because of developmental or learning disabilities, emotional problems, or, increasingly, infertility in adult women, although infertility affects a minority of women with Trisomy X. Many health professionals are unfamiliar with Trisomy X, and not inclined to recommend genetic testing for someone who does not look "syndromy." Many clinicians recommend that a prenatal diagnosis be confirmed after birth with additional testing to rule out the possibility of mosaicism, because girls who are mosaic and also have a Turner cell line, may have some of the health-related cardiac or gynecologic risks of females with Turner syndrome.

> *My doctor told us that if our unborn daughter had to have a genetic issue, Trisomy X is the one to have, so to speak. He said that many girls with this condition are completely normal, and that it is not physically noticeable. The issues that we could have might be with speech and motor delays, or learning disabilities. He did everything that he could to put our minds at ease. The doctor did have us speak with a genetic counselor, but no one encouraged us to terminate and we did not consider it.*

Symptoms, if they are present, are thought to occur because of the extra "dosing" involving gene activity on all three X chromosomes. In typical XX females, one of the X chromosomes is always inactivated. However, particular regions of the X chromosome, the pseudoautosomal regions, contain genes that govern the pairing between chromosomes during meiosis. These genes remain genetically active even when the rest of the chromosome is inactivated. These regions, then, contain genes that will provide, in a Trisomy X girl, a triple dose of genetic material.

One example is the SHOX gene, which is responsible for tall stature. A girl with Trisomy X has three activated copies, which probably explains why so many of these girls are quite tall. There is another group of genes on the X chromosome, and they may or may not be inactivated, which can account for more "triple" dosing in some females but not in others. This may account for the range in symptom expression from one female to the next in Trisomy X.

Babies with Trisomy X rarely have any physical signs of the condition other than mild hypotonia and subtle physical features including *clinodactyly* (curved little finger), *hypertelorism* (increased space between the eyes) or *epicanthal* eye folds, giving their eyes a somewhat rounded look. Occasionally, karyotyping is ordered because a child may be suspected of having Down syndrome, Trisomy 21, because of eye shape and low muscle tone.

While the risk of birth defects in Trisomy X is small, there is an increased incidence of genitourinary malformations (absence or malformation of a kidney, urinary tract, or reproductive organs), congenital hip dysplasia, and seizures. Children and adults frequently have hand tremors. Chronic constipation, perhaps associated with low muscle tone, affects a significant number of cases as does clinically significant gastroesophageal reflux. There have also been reports of congenital heart defects. In addition, the risk for development of auto-immune disorders, such as rheumatoid arthritis and lupus, is increased.

If developmental delays do occur, they generally affect speech-language and motor development. Babies with Trisomy X may walk independently later than usual, at 16 months, but still within what are considered normal limits. Babies may also show less stability in sitting, because of low muscle tone in the trunk, and they may have less manual dexterity than other children their age. Speech delays can be the result both of low muscle tone around the mouth, making it difficult for the toddler to form more difficult sounds, as well as dyspraxia of speech, which makes it difficult for the child to plan and initiate the movements and sound necessary for speech.

In some cases, the delay is pronounced and easily evident to a pediatrician in regular milestone screening. In others, the developmental lag is less severe, and parents and doctor take a "wait and see" approach to evaluation, particularly when there has not yet been a diagnosis. For girls who have been diagnosed prenatally and in infancy, any delay in meeting milestones should trigger an evaluation for early intervention services, as girls with Trisomy X can face a variety of educational and emotional challenges, and early intervention may help mitigate these problems later.

As with 47,XXY, IQ tends to be somewhat lower than for siblings, often by 15 to 20 points. Average IQ is about 85. The range of full scale IQs in various studies has been shown to be from about 55 to about 115. Most fall within the average/low-average range (75–90), but up to 10 percent may have mild intellectual disability. Verbal IQ is usually lower than performance IQ. Receptive language ability is also often greater than expressive language ability, and both oral and written expression can remain a problem throughout the lifetime, with relative weakness in word finding skills, sentence construction, and ability to narrate a story. There is also frequently difficulty with processing and understanding speech, and as school progresses, many girls will have difficulty with reading and spelling. Poor short term memory can amplify learning disabilities. In our study, more than two-thirds of girls had received early intervention services, and a similar percentage, a range of special education services from Section 504 accommodations to speech services to self-contained classrooms. The majority of girls, 54 percent, have Individualized Educational Plans (IEPs) in school.

Many girls with Trisomy X "hold their own" in elementary school and then find that with the increasing academic demands in middle school and high school, particularly for written expression and complex math skills, education accommodations are required to allow them to perform academically. Some of the other challenges that can affect school work include attention difficulties, executive functioning deficits and anxiety. A low frustration tolerance in many girls, and a tendency to emotional "meltdowns," can complicate instructional issues. In our survey, 23 percent had been diagnosed with ADHD and 33 percent with anxiety. Sensory processing difficulties are reported by a number of parents, including being overly sensitive to tags in garments, loud noises, tight "hugs," and other situations that make them uncomfortable and irritable.

> *She is a very generous person, with a funny sense of humor. She is smart, especially in language arts, she was an advanced reader from kindergarten on, and she writes well. She is also an excellent soccer player.*
>
> *The biggest challenge in school is her anxiety. Her learning disabilities are not severe, but she gets so upset if she has*

difficulty learning something, or if she gets less than a B on a paper. Although she does not need a smaller classroom and resource room to cope with her mild learning problems, she does need the smaller settings so that her anxiety doesn't get the better of her, choking off her ability to learn.

Parents commented on learning strategies that can work well with these girls, particularly in high school, that include decreasing distractions in the school setting with smaller classroom enrollment, use of individual tutoring, or switching to homeschooling for at least part of the day. Some families have had good experience with a self-contained classroom or a school that specializes in learning disabilities where distractions are minimized and teachers are focused on creating an atmosphere that maximizes learning potential.

As with boys who have XXY and XYY, maturity often lags chronological age in girls with Trisomy X. The deficits that girls experience include lack of facility with language to allow them to communicate effectively, as well as lack of social skills and executive functioning that are age-appropriate. This difficulty in "fitting in" and in being able to organize their lives and their schoolwork effectively contribute to the anxiety that many experience. Although fewer families were concerned that their daughters lack friendships, compared with families of boys with XXY and XYY, social relationships remain a problem for many girls. They can be too trusting, particularly of boys, and they can make poor choices in social situations. This deficit also contributes to family stress.

Difficulties in social situations are often exacerbated because Trisomy X girls have a tendency to be tall and may look older than their chronological age. At the same time, their functioning may appear to be immature. Families need to appreciate that school personnel and that the larger community may have unrealistic expectations for their daughters because of their appearance. The recommendation for coping with this satisfactorily is to acknowledge to the school that while she may be tall, she may actually have less maturity than her peers. She should not be pushed to perform at a level which she has not yet achieved. If she needs help with executive functioning as well as training in social skills, it is important to locate this assistance for her.

> *My greatest concern for my daughter is for the time when she is in high school and put in situations where her reasoning and judgment will be tested. I am concerned that she will look older due to her height, and yet her maturity is delayed compared with her peers. She will be faced with all the normal challenges of high school students without the benefit of the same level of maturity. I worry that she will harm herself, mentally or physically, due to bad decisions.*
>
> *I am concerned that when she goes to college, she could be a target. She is tall, beautiful and smart but she isn't world savvy, and someone could take advantage of her. Without having her parents around, she will need someone to check in on her socially and to help her organize herself academically. Otherwise, I think she has a bright future ahead of her.*

Although high school performance can be a challenge for many girls with Trisomy X, our survey found that of adults ages 18 and up, more than 80 percent were in college, working successfully, or occupied as homemakers. Although 38 percent reported having qualified for government disability benefits, most women receiving the benefits were also involved in furthering their education, or in working at least part-time. Adult independence may come later for these young women than for their XX sisters and peers. Families and schools need to take this into consideration, along with the fact that for many adults, earning a living wage may be limited, requiring them to depend on families or on government benefits in order to live independently in an apartment, for instance.

Women with Trisomy X usually have normal hormone levels and

most can become pregnant. Women with Trisomy X are at risk of premature ovarian failure (POF), which can lead to infertility. Some experience early or late *menarche* (first menstrual cycle) and others have abnormal menstrual cycles. There have been a small number of reports of women who have uterine or ovarian dysgenesis, in which the uterus and/or ovaries fail to develop, but this condition is rare.

The risk of a woman with non-mosaic Trisomy X transmitting the extra X chromosome to her offspring is small, less than 5 percent. Mosaicism with a Turner syndrome cell line (45,X) can increase the chances of transmission, however. Women with Trisomy X who are pregnant or contemplating pregnancy should consult with a genetic counselor to discuss these concerns.

> *I had a karyotype to figure out why my periods waned and then ceased. I was then told that I had premature ovarian failure, and Trisomy X. My chances of ever getting pregnant were now less than 1%.*
>
> *I remember having learning disabilities as a child. At the time of my 47,XXX, diagnosis, though, I did not believe that it had affected by life substantially. My son is a normal XY boy. I have a 6-year-old daughter, and she appears to be normal, although we have not had her tested.*

Most women with Trisomy X, however, go through menopause normally. Women with Trisomy X need to follow all recommendations for periodic sexual health visits, including regular Pap smears and breast exams.

It is clear that some adolescents and young adults with Trisomy X are developmentally delayed in terms of maturity, and are not ready as teens and young adults for social pressures, including those that they may encounter when dating young men. While Trisomy X is not a developmental disability, it can result in immaturity that makes her unable to recognize risky behavior and make appropriate choices.

Drug and alcohol use, and sexual activity present such situations. Peer pressure is often the reason that girls will engage in these activities, even when they would rather not. This is where parents need to establish open communication with their daughters, as well as "no fault" provisions so that the girl can call for a ride home, for instance, with no questions asked.

Similarly, girls need to know that they can approach their parents for emergency contraception or to talk with a gynecologist without creating an angry scene. Clear and unambiguous information about sexuality and reproduction is necessary for all young people with SCA, but especially for young women who tend to be tall and attractive and may be subject to pressure to engage in sexual activity before they are capable of making reasoned decisions about its emotional and physical consequences for them.

Many girls transition into adulthood with few problems. For others, additional support is necessary after high school in order to become established in adult life. The Transition to Adulthood section outlines many of the supports available, including government benefits, vocational training and preparation programs, special needs college services, and other services.

Tetrasomy X and Pentasomy X are rare conditions in females that are seen so infrequently that it is difficult to estimate the occurrence rates. The additional chromosomes are usually associated with intellectual disability, although there are girls and women with these conditions who have IQs in the low normal range. In general, each additional X chromosome decreases the IQ relative to siblings by approximately 15 points. Girls and women as a group with Tetrasomy X generally experience less disability than those with Pentasomy X, but that is not always the case with individuals

There is significant variation for both conditions from one female to another, although some general statements regarding the phenotypes can be made. The majority of the girls can be described as pleasant and affectionate although a bit shy, with a good sense of humor. They may become easily frustrated, however, and be prone to emotional outbursts. There is frequently some mild facial dysmorphia that may include features such as epicanthal eye folds, a flat nasal bridge, hypertelorism (wide space between eyes), midface hypoplasia (flattened facial appearance). Sometimes there may be facial asymmetry or unusual ear placement and shape. They may have nystigmus (uncontrolled eye movements) or strabismus (lazy eye). They may also have minor mouth deformities, high palates or cleft palates, and distinct over- or under-bites. Girls with Pentasomy X tend to have more pronounced facial features, which can also include a short, broad neck, and some girls with Pentasomy X have microcephaly, or a head circumference in the lowest percentiles, indicating a small brain and significant intellectual disability.

Low birthweights have been reported along with obstetrical complications including heart problems during delivery and respiratory problems in the immediate neonatal period. Girls with these conditions will often have additional skeletal and motor abnormalities including significant hypotonia, congenital torticollis, clinodactyly, congenital hip dysplasia, palmer creases (a straight line crease across the palm of the hands, often indicative of a genetic disorder). There can be somewhat odd angulation of linbs, radioulnar synostosis, and general joint laxity. Again, the number and severity of physical signs tends to increase with Pentasomy X.

> *My sister is the most resilient person I've ever met. She has been through more medical issues than ten people combined, and yet she doesn't let it get her down. She also possesses an innocence that is a constant reminder to the rest of us that people should look at the world the way she does. My biggest concern other than her health is her quality of life. She straddles the fence of not being so handicapped that she is helpless, but cognitively, she has only the grasp of the world of a child. As a 28-year-old that is a dangerous combination. And she is so trusting.*

There are a number of medical complications associated with Tetrasomy X and Pentasomy X. Seizures and abnormal EEGs are not uncommon as are congenital heart defects. Respiratory difficulties including asthma and recurrent pneumonia and bronchitis are reported. Although the genitalia appear to be normal, only about fifty percent of these girls undergo puberty normally with full development of secondary sexual characteristics. Menstrual irregularities and early menopause are common. Some girls have an abnormally developed uterus and ovaries. A number require estrogen therapy to prevent osteoporosis and achieve breast development. Most of the women have problems with their dental enamel, causing significant decay, and their jaw problems often require extensive orthodontia.

Developmental problems include late walking, poor fine and gross motor skills and delayed speech. Attention deficits are common, along with significant learning disabilities. Girls and women can have behavioral difficulties associated with frustration and difficulties in communicating clearly. There can be psychiatric problems associated with the conditions including anxiety, depression and occasionally, psychosis. There are also reports of young women doing fairly well in school and being able to attend vocational programs or college. Many can work at least part-time, although nearly all will access government benefits for persons with developmental disabilities, and will require some degree of supervision throughout their lives.

Psychosocial Considerations in Sex Chromosome Aneuploid Conditions

I am a social worker and not trained in psychology. While numerous articles on the psychology of individuals with SCA are available, I have seen no written material describing how individuals with SCA fit within their family systems and the community, nor materials guiding families and individuals affected by one of the SCAs in navigating those systems. This section seeks to outline issues involved with a lifespan approach to these concerns. Because there is substantial overlap among KS, Trisomy X, and 47,XYY, in psychosocial domains, the discussion here is general and does not focus on the specific differences in testing scores among SCA groups, for instance, that an academic paper might. Rather, this section provides an overview of how SCA may affect an individual in a particular area, such as "social skills." It also suggests an approach to coping strategies for the affected individuals as well as their family members and other people of significance in their lives.

It cannot be repeated too often that there is substantial phenotypic variation within SCA groups and among all individuals with supernumerary X and Y chromosomes. Some individuals have only the mildest of psychosocial functioning difficulty in a few areas, while some have significant difficulty in a majority of areas. This overview is meant to point readers in the direction of identifying areas where they may wish to explore interventions and professional assistance.

We know that, in general, people with additional X chromosomes will have **cognitive abilities** that may be somewhat lower than siblings, typically 10–20 IQ points less per extra X chromosome. It is not as clear by how much an extra Y chromosome affects IQ relative to siblings. While intellectual disability is not common, it is more frequently seen in individuals with SCA, particularly those who have variations that include 48 and 49 chromosomes, rather than the trisomy conditions. This is "group" data, however, and an individual is not a group. Similarly, while the **personalities** of 47,XXY, boys and 47,XXX, girls may be somewhat more reserved than average, this is also group data, and within the group there will be those who are outgoing and not the least bit shy.

Individuals with SCA and their families need to have the best picture of cognitive functioning, language skills, and other psychosocial characteristics possible, including an assessment of strengths and weaknesses. People with SCA need to be seen as unique, with highly individualized abilities as well as challenges. At several critical junctures during the early life of an individual with SCA, it is advantageous to have *neuropsychological* testing done to evaluate exactly how the individual functions on a variety of cognitive and personality tests. This testing can be used to design specific interventions in school age children, and once a child reaches adulthood, to help in choosing postsecondary education options and to help assist in making vocational decisions. Sometimes, it can also be used as supporting material to access government assistance programs, such as vocational rehabilitation services or income support programs, including Supplemental Security Income (SSI) or Social Security Disability Income (SSDI). Neuropsychological testing can also help to guide therapists. Most important, it gives the person and the family a very individualized view of his or her strengths and weaknesses.

Neuropsychological testing should be performed by a doctoral level psychologist who has specialized in psychometrics and diagnosis. School districts will sometimes perform such testing in-house, but while this will provide basic information on intelligence and learning potential, it probably is not the comprehensive and independent overview of the individual that he desires or that his or her family would want.

Testing may take place over several days and often requires 10–15 hours to complete. The neuropsychologist will follow this with a session to explain the findings fully, as well as providing a comprehensive written report. For families looking for special education services, this really represents the "gold standard." For individuals who may want vocational counseling and services, special accommodations in college or in the workplace, and realistic guidance in planning their futures, high quality neuropsychological testing is critical.

This testing can be expensive, typically costing at least $150 per hour. Many insurance companies may not cover its cost. Insurers, however, are much more likely to cover the testing if it is justified with the medical diagnosis of a genetic disorder associated with neurological problems.

It is important to see the person with SCA as an individual, and not solely as a member of a group of persons with a particular phenotype, with personality and abilities predetermined by his or her extra chromosome(s). It is equally important to understand that while cognitive and social functioning as a child can help to predict how that child performs as an adult, there may be rather striking changes between the personality and cognitive abilities of a person in childhood and those of the same person well into adulthood.

Particularly for those who have significant challenges with language, and therefore with socialization and academic performance during school years, adulthood often offers freedom from various pressures, and from being surrounded by what they perceive as children to be constant failure. A number of our adults in the survey noted that school years had been unhappy, because they did not do well academically, and because they were subject to teasing because of their lack of confidence, lack of athletic abilities and, for men with KS, lack of the typical male physique. Adulthood was far more satisfying for many of the adults surveyed, whether they had KS, Trisomy X, or 47,XYY. We do not have a great deal of valid, non-biased research on adults with SCA. Much of the high-quality research includes longitudinal studies done on young children that followed them into the teens, but not many studies have continued into adulthood.

Researchers now have available the MRI as a tool with which to measure and map the various regions of the brain in SCA. They can also observe how and where the brain is functioning during cognitive tasks, which is called *functional MRI, or fMRI.* A number of these studies have been done over the past two decades with children and adults with SCA. The results may lead to more specific educational and behavioral or psychological interventions in the future to address the impact of genetics as well as hormone levels on brain development and cognitive and emotional functioning. Currently, however, what we know about the relationship between brain differences and extra X and Y chromosomes is still fairly limited. The studies, because of the expense and the logistical difficulties of enrolling a large enough sample for research imaging, are not large enough yet to provide conclusive answers.

With 47,XYY, subjects, only one small study has been done, and no differences in brain volume compared with controls were found. In subjects with KS, MRI studies have shown a reduction in brain volume compared with control subjects. In the subjects studied, however, having a lower brain volume was not necessarily predictive of lower IQ, so the impact of reduced brain volume is probably related to a number of measures of cognitive functioning, not just IQ. There is some evidence that males with KS process language differently, perhaps because of differences in the size of brain lobes as well as activity levels of right and left hemispheres, compared with controls. The amygdala, which helps to control emotion, also appears to be reduced in volume in males with KS, but this was also not shown to be correlated with increased emotional distress in the individuals studied.

There is also one very small MRI study that compares brain structure and volume of men treated with testosterone with men who have not received testosterone treatment. This appears to show an increase in the volume of some brain structures for men who have used testosterone when compared to men who have not. Because of the small sample size, the study's statistical power is weak.

MRI studies in females with Trisomy X showed findings that were similar to those of males with KS, so it does appear that an extra X chromosome reduces brain volume. The studies of individuals with trisomy SCA, however, are too small to provide the statistical power to conclude that particular differences in volume or processing relative to control subjects has any particular cognitive, language processing or emotional result. We need more and larger studies to draw more firm conclusions about the impact of an extra X chromosome.

It has been even more difficult to run statistically significant MRI studies of individuals with 48- and 49-chromosome SCA variations. In individuals with SCA variations, there are a few case reports of MRI studies as well as one larger study of males with 48,XXYY. Although a number of the studies show individual gross abnormalities with lowered brain volume and abnormal brain structure, as well as abnormalities in the white and grey matter making up the brain, there are no clear conclusions that can be drawn at this time.

Social skills and communication in relationships are major challenges noted by both adults with SCA and parents of children and adults with SCA. Some impairment not only in the use of language but also in "reading" behavior affects the majority of individuals with SCA, at every age. Social skills and communication contribute to being accepted in the classroom and on the playground, and later in early adulthood in the workplace as well as in forming intimate relationships. Poor social skills can further decrease self-esteem in children already struggling with poor academic performance. And for young adults with learning disabilities, success on the job is often determined more by the ability to "get along" with supervisors and coworkers, than it is by being able to do the tasks of the job competently.

While many young children with SCA have language delays, and can have language-based learning disabilities, it isn't enough for them to finally acquire functional language, to be able to express themselves reasonably well, and to learn to read and write. For those with SCA, the more hidden communication handicaps stem from difficulties, often life-long, in social communications. Social communications involve verbal and non-verbal behaviors that make up social interactions. They include the importance of eye contact during conversation, making "small talk" to break the ice with a stranger, and learning to read subtle cues on the part of the other person that he wants to change the topic. A child who lacks social skills may have great difficulty making friends at school, and an adult may be unable to build a network of supportive friends as he grows older, as well as having a more difficult time in finding a close partner with whom he can have a romantic relationship.

Answers to the survey told me that adults with SCA can suffer loneliness, and that they often seem to realize that their loneliness may be the result of having communication difficulties that make social interaction difficult. This can cause or exacerbate emotional difficulties. Adults told me that they knew that they might be seen as somewhat more reserved than normal or a bit shy, but that the problem isn't shyness. It is lack of social ability to connect meaningfully with others. For many adults, who have tried hard to develop social skills on which they can build confidence, relationships have become easier. With this easing of ability to relate to other people, they have built small networks of support, which have made their lives more satisfying.

Parents who see their children struggling with loneliness, or with bullying in school—a cruel form of ostracizing people with learning and behavioral differences—may be looking for a treatment for social skill deficits. There is quite a bit of emphasis on social skills training for children on the autism spectrum, but the techniques are also applicable to children who are affected by ADHD, non-verbal learning disabilities, and also SCA.

> *Her judgment in groups concerns me. She wants everyone to like her and she doesn't seem to yet to have the skills to cope with bullies or with general "meanness." We work a lot with her on her sense of self-worth and on her confidence in group settings.*

Social skills training can be done individually or in groups. It can have a language-based emphasis, and be provided by a speech therapist, or it can be provided by therapists or specially trained special education teachers. It may focus on elementary concepts, providing children with "scripts" for dealing with certain situations, like meeting a new person, or ordering food at a restaurant. More advanced training will focus on reading subtle and non-verbal cues.

When looking for social skills training for a school-age child, it is most beneficial if the child can be involved in classes and experiences that also include typically developing peers. It also is more effective if the groups allow for generalization of what is learned in the group to real situations in the classroom or in social settings outside of school. Social skills training often involves "homework" given out for practice during the week. Parents of children involved in social skills training should also request that they receive parent training in reinforcing the lessons of the training sessions, so that they can help their children to apply skills in everyday life. Another methodology that can be used to teach social skills and appropriate behavior in a number of different situation is the "social story" technique pioneered by Carol Gray, whose website and published materials provide clear directions to parents and teachers.

Finding appropriate social skills training for adults is more difficult. An adult who feels that he or she is missing the level of skills necessary for effective social communication may more easily find communication therapy one-on-one with a speech therapist. Individual communication skills therapy may also be useful for older children and adolescents, especially if they do not "fit" well in social skills groups aimed at more obviously disabled children. The speech therapist will focus on speech pragmatics which is the use of language and conversation for communication and socialization. The focus of such therapy is often on relating stories in an organized manner, increasing the variety of language used to communicate, learning to "converse" and to take the perspective of the other partners in the conversation, and avoiding inappropriate topics or unrelated subjects when having a conversation.

An additional concern for individuals with extra X and Y chromosomes is **executive functioning.** Executive skills are the cognitive activities that allow for coordination of all goal-directed behaviors that accomplish particular tasks. Executive functions include the ability to initiate activities, monitor and change behavior when necessary, anticipate outcomes, and adapt to changing situations. It also includes the ability to inhibit or stop behaviors when that is necessary, controlling impulses that could lead to negative outcomes.

One example might be shopping for food for a meal. It requires sequencing the steps needed to buy, prepare and cook, and making certain that the steps are accomplished before the time that the meal is needed such as dinnertime. Time management is an important consideration here, as is checking before shopping that the funds are present, either in cash or in the form of credit or debit card or food stamps, to purchase the food.

A planning process takes place, either on paper or "on the run" on entering the grocery store, to determine what ingredients need to be purchased. This includes memory work to determine whether some of the necessary ingredients such as spices, cooking oil, salad dressing, or other items are already available at home in the kitchen. The shopping trip involves selection of ingredients, comparing prices, calculating needed quantities, and finally determining that the shopping list is complete. There are appropriate behaviors in the checkout line that need to be coordinated. Throughout the entire process, the individual has to focus his attention on the tasks, and manage his or her ability to resist distractions.

The process of managing all of these tasks and behaviors constitutes executive functioning. If executive functioning is faulty, an individual with perfectly normal intelligence, capable of performing all of the tasks individually, can fail to orchestrate the entire process smoothly. Key ingredients are forgotten, or he returns home two hours after dinnertime, or he forgets that he had only enough money in his food stamp account to purchase $20.00 worth of groceries, not the $50.00 that he processed through the checkout line. If he lacks appropriate executive functioning, he will discover that he has made a mess of the shopping expedition, which further frustrates him. His lack of impulse control, which is also an executive functioning deficit, may make him unable to avoid yelling at the cashier when he discovers that he can't pay for his purchases. And he will probably be unable to problem-solve his way out of his dilemma independently, perhaps storming out of the grocery store, and arriving home empty-handed.

The size and perhaps the structures involving the frontal lobes of the brain govern the processes needed for planning, flexibility, organization and self-monitoring. In individuals with SCA, the frontal lobes may not function optimally to control these behaviors. Developing executive functioning is a trial and error process in typically developing individuals. In individuals with SCA, it may require particular training techniques to learn these skills as well as strategies to compensate for deficits in working memory capacity and ability to focus attention on tasks. Schools often do well with helping children compensate for specific learning disabilities but fail to adopt strategies that address executive functioning deficits. With adults with SCA, we often see relatively high-functioning individuals who struggle with organizing many aspects of their everyday lives because no one has addressed their issues of executive functioning.

> *One thing that makes a world of difference for my daughter is that she understand very clearly what is being asked of her and exactly what is expected. She cannot "read between the lines." We really need to spell out the process of doing something line by line. Unfortunately, she does not always feel comfortable telling others that she doesn't understand what someone is telling her to do, or when she does not understand a word.*
>
> *I believe that I have some symptoms of autism spectrum*

disorder, like sensory processing disorder. I also have anxiety that results from changes in plans that I did not expect or when I am told to do something without adequate time to prepare. I have adapted, but it has taken a lot of time and patience. I now work for a company that provides waiver services to individuals who have intellectual or developmental disabilities. They seem to understand the approach that I need to do a job well.

After finding out that I have XXY, I told many of my closest friends and family. I am very open to discussing the topic and its impact on my ability to function. I feel that by opening up to people and letting them know how to work best with me, it has made a direct positive effect on my life.

Addressing these problems requires the recognition that the individual may be overwhelmed with the challenge of managing his activities. He or she is not lazy, but rather cannot initiate an activity, or is reluctant to try because past failures are associated with negative consequences. Another party such as a family member or a life skills trainer or a tutor must modify the activity and help him to adopt new and more functional techniques of approaching multi-faceted tasks.

If working with a young adult who cannot seem to accomplish "anything" during the day, it helps to set up a routine for his or her day, week and month. A visual schedule in the form of a wall planner is very useful in accomplishing this. A smart phone that can display the schedule as well as beep to alert him or her to appointments is also a powerful tool for helping with time management. Both wall calendar and a calendar that can be carried in the phone will provide continuous reminders of scheduled activities. Don't expect a young person to manage this calendar independently at first. It may need setup and maintenance by another party initially who helps the individual to begin taking responsibility for it in stages. It is also useful to provide a prominently located clock in each room that the person occupies so that he can become accustomed to seeing and checking the time. A digital clock works best for many teens and young adults with SCA.

The reader may be thinking at this point that executive functioning deficits sound an awful lot like the difficulties of attention deficit disorder, or ADHD, with or without the hyperactivity. Many families and adults report that ADHD has been diagnosed in individuals with SCA, and ADHD is considered to be one of the conditions that is frequently co-morbid with extra X and Y chromosomes. In our survey, the numbers exceeded 50 percent. There is substantial overlap in the time and activity management difficulties experienced by those with ADHD, with non-verbal learning disabilities, and by those with executive functioning deficits.

Although psychologists have very specific definitions and criteria for diagnosis of each problem, for the person suffering the consequences of this disorganization, it doesn't really matter what it is called, because the strategies that can be helpful are quite similar. In addition to creating routines and providing the individual with both wall (large visual) and smart phone calendars, the following measures can not only help cope with executive functioning deficits, but will also provide the experience that can help him or her learn to cope more independently in the long term.

Working memory is frequently poor in SCA, creating problems with following multi-step directions, holding a thought, and creating and sticking to a plan. A strategy for coping with poor working memory is to reduce distractions when being given directions or when working on a problem, to do the task right away, to write out reminders and detailed instructions. This can help to commit facts and events to long-term memory.

Starting and finishing tasks is often a weak point for persons with SCA. They are poor at initiating tasks, often because of fear engendered by previous failures, so they procrastinate. They may feel guilty about procrastinating, and they may feel dread because failure to start is yet another failure. For those who do start, yet lack the ability to direct themselves to complete a good-quality project, the task may remain unfinished—more reason for their parents, supervisors and others to get irritated with them. It helps to have a non-judgmental tutor, coach or other party work with the individual to set realistic mini-deadlines, and reward the person for each mini-deadline met until the project is complete.

Planning behavior is often absent in people with SCA. They have difficulty in carefully thinking through the consequences of their behavior on the future. They need to be coached to stop and consider how an activity will affect their futures. (Spray-painting graffiti may seem fun right now but it involves potential involvement in the criminal justice system.) Responsible decision-making should be specifically rewarded.

Emotional self-control may be another area that is lacking in the person with SCA. People with SCA may display strong reactions that come and go quickly and that appear to be over-reactions to fairly ordinary events. These emotions can cause the person to behave spontaneously and without thinking of the consequences. The person with SCA is then seen as immature and impulsive. People can be trained to step back from a situation before reacting, and if they do overreact, they can apologize. Helping a person who is already an adult to gain control over emotional outbursts often requires the intervention of a professional from outside the family.

Families and individuals may find assistance with developing executive functioning in adolescents and adults with SCA through coaches who work with individuals with ADHD and Asperger syndrome. The problems caused by executive functioning deficits are often at the center of family tension, anger and guilt. Family members may need some assistance from professionals to help them adopt more productive strategies with their adolescent and adult members. It is sometimes impossible to do this without the assistance of outside parties whose relations with the person with SCA are not so bound up with negative emotions. Coaches can be located by contacting local chapters of CHADD (Children and Adults with Attention Deficit-Hyperactivity

Disorder), www.chadd.org or local Asperger syndrome organizations, including www.grasp.org.

Sometimes executive functioning difficulties are accompanied by ADHD, and sometimes not. It appears that executive functioning difficulties in KS are more pronounced if the individual also has a diagnosis of ADHD. If it seems that a child or an adult may meet the criteria for ADHD because of distractibility, poor time management and impulsivity, it is worth a consultation, but it should be with a psychiatrist or psychologist (or developmental pediatrician) who is skilled at diagnosing and treating ADHD.

Medication may or may not be useful, particularly for situations, like school or work, where an individual must maintain focus for a period of several hours. There are various well-proven measures, such as Connors scales, that can help to determine if medication can help or is making a measurable difference. Medication is unlikely to help much, however, unless attention is also made to behavioral and environmental strategies that help the child or adult to build executive functioning skills.

For families of children and adolescents, particularly, **emotional dysregulation** can lead to angry outbursts, tantrums, and "meltdowns." All children, whether typically developing or with neuro-developmental delays, will have these episodes. When they become disruptive of family life and threaten to impact negatively a child's education, they need to be addressed by professionals. It helps to remember that the child has an immature response system to handle emotions that overwhelm him or her. When a meltdown occurs, the parent has to remain in control.

Initially, determine whether this is a manipulative tantrum or is the result of emotions running out of control in the child. If he is having a tantrum because he wants to watch another hour of TV, it is important not to give in but simply to put him in "time out" until he can quiet himself. Reactions to manipulative tantrums have to be consistent. The parent needs to make certain that the tantrum does not turn into a tool that trains the parent to "give in."

If the parent determines, however, that the child is overwhelmed with fatigue or with an emotional response that he can't control, then the parent or the teacher needs to take control for him. Talk as calmly as possible and take him to a quiet place, even if it means leaving the grocery store for a car. There are many techniques available in books and online for helping the overwhelmed child to come out of a meltdown. Read some of this material and adopt techniques that you find are helpful, and try to develop relaxation methods for you and your child to gain control over the situation. If necessary, find a child psychologist who can help you learn behavioral techniques to manage a child's anger and outbursts and to de-escalate the situation.

It may also be useful to consult an occupational therapist about methods for modifying the child's environment if sensory issues are a factor in his emotional response. Children with SCA can have over-sensitivity to things like buzzing fluorescent lights or scratchy fabrics. They can also have so much difficulty with coordination and motor skills to perform school work or activities of daily living, such as getting dressed, that emotional outbursts may result. Occupational therapists are trained to identify sensory issues and frustrations borne of motor skill difficulties and heightened sensitivies, and can help you to make adaptations than can minimize behavioral difficulties.

> *Anxiety and frustration are by far his greatest issues, and this sometimes looks like anger. Martial arts have given him confidence in his ability to defend himself if someone is sarcastic or rude to him, and it has also given him self-control so that his reaction is only so much as the situation requires. As parents, we encourage him to take a step back and walk away before he loses his cool when he is frustrated. This is a work in progress but huge changes have been made in the last five years. We have been teaching him coping skills and appropriate interpersonal skills since early childhood.*

For individuals who get all the way to adulthood without being able to regulate their emotional behavior successfully, this can lead to job loss and damaged relationships with family. These adults or their caregivers/advocates will need to find therapists and coaches who can help them to develop control. Emotional dysregulation in adults is often a complex brew of executive functioning deficits combined with anxiety and depression, with one problem feeding off another. The dysregulation can worsen and can contribute to more serious psychiatric difficulty. The individual knows at some level that his angry outbursts are driving away the very people who can help him as well as making it difficult to build relationships and hold a job.

Many young adults with SCA are stuck in a pattern of anger at their parents as they try to navigate early adulthood with the maturity level of someone in the mid-teens. It can be tough for the parents, who love them dearly, to put up with negative behavior as they try to assist them in transitioning to independence, which usually means becoming largely self-supporting through work as well as leaving home and establishing an independent household. And it can also be a challenge for life coaches or therapists who are hired to work with these individuals, because they will also have anger directed at them. Parents or others working with the individual who has SCA may need to find therapists and life coaches who are familiar with high-functioning developmental disorders such as Asperger syndrome. It also helps to make certain that the therapist or life coach understands the sorts of executive functioning, learning, social and other challenges that may underlie the anger of the individual with SCA.

Beyond executive functioning deficits, emotional dysregulation, and attention disorders, other **psychiatric difficulties** are known to be comorbid with SCA. The extent of the risk has been measured as high as six to eight times that of the general population for all SCA groups while more recent studies using tighter and more detailed diagnostic standards show a lower risk, and more specifically identify the disorders. We do know that both children and adults are at heightened risk for anxiety and mood disorders, including depression, panic disorders, and phobias.

With the caveat that our survey is of self-reported diagnosis, and that our survey is not on a scientifically determined sample, it should be noted that adults with KS and Trisomy X reported that 68 percent had suffered from either anxiety or depression. Many included statements that they had coped with varying anxiety and depression throughout their lifetimes. They viewed this as a result of the life stresses of learning and communication disabilities. Men with KS stated that the knowledge that they were infertile contributed to their sadness. A number also said that once they were treated with testosterone, much of their anxiety and depression resolved.

It is also known that SCA may affect the size of the amygdala, and that this, in turn, may negatively impact emotional regulation, and contribute to mood disorder. Four percent of these adults reported a diagnosis of bipolar disorder. Women with Trisomy X and men with KS reported a rate of substance abuse at any time in the past or currently of 9 percent, which is roughly equal to the national average in the United States for substance abuse. Many adults who reported substance abuse stated that this was an attempt to self-medicate for anxiety and depression.

For KS males and those with KS variations of all ages in our survey, the rate of anxiety and depression was reported to be 48 percent and the rate of bipolar disorder, 3 percent. Five percent reported a diagnosis of psychotic disorder.

For females with Trisomy, Tetrasomy and Pentasomy X of all ages, the rate of anxiety and depression was reported at 45 percent with bipolar disorder reported at 4 percent. Psychotic disorders were reported at 5 percent.

> *He already experiences bouts of depression and anxiety, and he has such a disturbing fear of failure that he will not even attempt a task if he believes that he won't be able to complete*

it perfectly. In addition to struggling with learning issues and with social difficulties in school, mental health is a big challenge for us.

The responses for all ages of males with 47,XYY, reported an anxiety and depression rate of 53 percent; a rate of bipolar disorder of 13 percent; and a rate of psychotic disorder of 6 percent. It should be noted that the rate of autism spectrum diagnosis was 32 percent for those with 47,XYY, while it was much lower, about 6 percent, for both Trisomy X and 47,XXY.

Because this was not a scientific survey, no conclusions regarding psychiatric risk can be made. In the United States, it is estimated that at any time 9.5 percent of adults are suffering from depression. I did not ask the same question in the survey, so we do not know how many people with SCA are suffering from depression at a given time. What the survey does tell us, however, is that psychiatric co-morbidity is a serious concern for those with SCA. Brain structure, genetic dosing effects, and hormonal factors are probably at work, with the risk heightened because of the stresses of struggling with learning disabilities. A number of adults and parents noted that bullying is a factor in depression and anxiety in childhood and that this can stretch into affecting mood in adulthood.

Adults who reported, however, are likely to speak of their depression as being something that happened "in the past." Many tell about moving on beyond their emotional difficulties after a process of accepting their limitations and learning to embrace their differences. Depression and anxiety can and do resolve, particularly when there are important situational contributions, such as developmental delay along with a more extended period required to reach adult maturity. Adolescence and young adulthood can be very difficult for some in this population. For most, becoming established as an independently functioning adult, although it may happen somewhat later than for typically developing siblings and peers, leads to improved emotional functioning.

Signs of psychiatric disorders, particularly the more subtle signs of sadness and irritability in children and adults, need to be paid careful attention. My husband and I did not know when John was young that he was at increased risk for anxiety and depression. In fact, when he did appear to have major depression in elementary school and became suicidal, we did not fully realize his level of depression until he drew a detailed map of where and how he would commit suicide, along with plans for setting off a bomb at his school. In hindsight, we should have removed him from school before this incident happened instead of encouraging him to go each day even though we knew he was increasingly and painfully anxious. When he finally made so overt a suicide threat, we were told that he could not return to the elementary school. The results of that episode followed him throughout his school years, and he was never able to be mainstreamed successfully after that. Maturity, mood stabilizers, and testosterone treatment have caused him to become much more stable as an adult, but I know that psychiatric disorder in childhood is a searing experience for both the child and the parents.

Prevention of psychiatric disability in this population starts with providing as good a home life as possible, along with high-quality schooling where bullying is not tolerated. Children with SCA need to be sheltered somewhat from undue stresses at school. They may already have considerable stress because of difficulty learning and lack of social skills. If they are being bullied, and if the school is not responsive to their needs, it is not a "safe" place for them. For many parents, this has meant abandoning public education after trying numerous measures to get the system to work for their children. Some choose to place their child in a private school that can provide smaller classrooms and more flexibility in meeting their child's learning and social needs. An increasing number of parents posting on the listserves have turned to homeschooling, with the many online supports that are available today. Parents need to try to provide their children with as many opportunities for success as possible. They also need to realize that even with doing everything "right," anxiety, depression, or a more serious psychiatric disorder may develop in their child. In that case, they should make every effort to avoid denying the situation, and seek competent mental health services.

For adults with SCA, it helps immeasurably to avoid substance abuse, which can exacerbate mood disorders. Building strong relationships with a few good friends is important, as is becoming established in a career. If emotional problems become a barrier to successfully pursuing education, a career, or relationships, then help should be sought. Medication can help to make someone "feel" much better, and it can be essential to maintaining emotional stability. But it is more effective if it is accompanied by appropriate psychotherapy.

For relatively high-functioning adults with developmental issues, whether they have learning disabilities or executive functioning challenges, *cognitive behavioral therapy (CBT)*, is particularly useful. CBT has a focus on the patient's belief system, and teaches the patient to adopt a new way of thinking about and reacting toward issues. It is particularly useful for those who have low self-esteem, and have a constant flow of negative thoughts toward themselves and others. CBT is generally time-limited and problem-focused. It requires that the person in therapy to commit to "homework" and to regular weekly visits to measure progress toward goals. There are many effective variations on CBT, including dialectical behavioral therapy and rational emotive therapy. It often is not so much the actual methodology that helps as it is a trusting relationship with a therapist who can help the client to see how to break out of old patterns of thinking, and adopt new and more effective behaviors.

Educational Recommendations for Individuals with SCA

The range of educational performance of individuals with extra X and Y chromosomes is quite broad. About one-third of individuals with trisomy SCA do not need any special assistance in school, and do not struggle with reading, math, or other subjects. But for the other two-thirds of those with trisomy conditions, and for nearly all of the children with 48 and 49 chromosomes, special attention must be given to educational interventions that range from simple environmental modifications in the classroom to reduce distractions, to placement in a small, self-contained classroom with highly individualized instruction.

It is impossible to generalize about educational needs of this population. This section, however, explains the organization of special education services in the United States: early intervention services covering birth to 3 years; preschool education for ages 3–5; and school-age services for children attending kindergarten through high school. High school generally ends at age 18, but for special education students, public education can extend to age 21, although this is reserved for children with the most severe disabilities. In addition, the section provides some educational strategies that appear to be effective for a number of children with SCA. Readers from other countries will have to adapt this material to their own educational institutions.

The Education of All Handicapped Children Act of 1975 mandated a free and appropriate education for children with disabilities. The law was strengthened and reauthorized in 2004 as the Individuals with Disabilities Education Act, or IDEA. In 1986, Public Law 99–457 was passed which entitled all children with disabilities ages birth to age 5 to special education and therapeutic services. Many countries around the world have passed and follow similar legislation regarding children with disabilities. Regardless of the country in which they live, parents of children identified with extra X and Y chromosomes are likely to come into contact with these systems, and to need to learn the system of acronyms for the assessments, documents and systems that will provide access to these services for their children. This chapter provides a basic outline of services in order to give parents an overview of the system at various stages in a child's or young adult's education and training.

For children ages birth to age 3, the service delivery system in most states is the Early Intervention system. It is authorized by the **Early Intervention Program** for Infants and Toddlers, Part C of IDEA. (For additional information about the program and to find information about services in each individual state, visit the National Early Childhood Technical Assistance Center, www.nectac.org.) Multidisciplinary services including speech-language services, occupational therapy and physical therapy are available. Eligibility standards vary but all states are required to provide early intervention for children with established conditions that are associated with intellectual disability or developmental delays. They are also required to serve children with sufficient developmental delay, regardless of diagnosis of an "established condition."

The dilemma here is that so many children with SCA initially have mild developmental delays which may not alone qualify them for early intervention services. In addition, many evaluators may be unfamiliar with SCA. It may be necessary to have the child's pediatrician brief the evaluation team on the developmental trajectory of children with SCA, including the fact that the combined effect of language, motor skill and social impairments place the child at significant risk of more severe delay as he becomes older. It is also helpful if the pediatrician can convince the Early Intervention team to consider SCA to be an "established condition," as it is in some states.

Our state 0–3 Year program is very good. We had qualified therapists who produced good results in reducing his speech and motor delays. It was nice to be able to receive these services at home. Our son began receiving services at 4 months and continued until he moved into the school system at age 3. Our son's IEP is based on his medical condition, which is helpful since it would be difficult to qualify him on delay alone because he isn't in the "bottom 10 percent." He has been attending a special needs preschool part-time through the school system, as well as a community-based preschool where he is mainstreamed with typically developing kids. This should prepare him well for kindergarten, while the special needs preschool provides the therapies that he needs.

It took two tries, but she was not developmentally delayed "enough" to qualify until her second birthday. The first year of services was great. When she was three, parents were no longer included and also provided training in reinforcing the services, so it was no longer so helpful. At that point, we started private speech therapy in addition, and this did wonders for her progress.

Assessments for EI must include an evaluation by professionals from at least two disciplines. The assessment must cover the child's functioning in the areas of cognition, speech-language and communication, motor and physical development, adaptive behavior, and socio-emotional development. A written Individualized Family Service Plan (IFSP) is developed by the parents and evaluators that describe the EI services to be provided, along with the setting for service provision. Because there is a priority placed on services provided in the child's "natural environment," services are often home-based and delivered by therapists who travel to the child's home or to his or her daycare provider. The IFSP should be reviewed at least once per year or more often if there are significant developmental issues to consider.

If a child is considered ineligible for EI services, the diagnosed condition of SCA often makes speech therapy, OT and PT reimbursable by insurance, as long as a pediatrician or other medical professional prescribes the services. Because developmental delay may become more pronounced as a child gets older, it is worth continuing to monitor the child's progress with his or her pediatrician, and to request a re-evaluation if indicated. This section does not make any general statements on what either EI or preschool services should entail. Children with SCA are highly individual, and the child's needs for services should drive the therapies that are provided.

Children usually transition from EI services to **preschool special education services** (Part B of the IDEA) provided through the public school district at age three. The child's services are then governed by an IEP, or Individualized Education Program. The eligibility categories also change, and children who may have been qualified for EI as "developmentally delayed" may no longer qualify, because they are not considered to be sufficiently delayed to need services. In this case, the family may want to change the preschooler's eligibility category to "other health impaired," which requires an overall assessment of the medical condition's impact on the child's educational needs.

For children who do not qualify for preschool special education, allow a developmental pediatrician to guide you in deciding whether or not to obtain speech, OT or PT services privately. Introducing the child to part-time preschool is a good idea so that he or she can interact with other children in a group setting and become accustomed to a classroom prior to entering kindergarten.

My son's preschool teacher took great interest in him. With her help, I was able to have him attend preschool for another year. He receives speech and occupational therapy which were important in helping him to acquire skills that he will need for kindergarten, and which he did not yet have at age 5. In addition, the special education teachers were the ones who pushed for further testing, including genetic testing, which is how we found that he has Klinefelter syndrome.

The preschool teacher can help parents to determine if there are any areas of developmental concern that should be addressed before the child starts kindergarten. Whether to start a child in kindergarten at age five, or to wait for an additional year until the child is six, is an individual decision for parents to make. In favor of waiting until the child is six is the fact that many children with SCA are at least slightly behind in both motor and social skills, and often in speech-language skills, as well. The extra year of maturity may make them better able to compete with peers. On the downside, children with extra X and Y chromosomes may be tall for their age, and therefore will both appear and be chronologically older than many of their classmates if they begin school at age 6.

When children enter **elementary school**, they will usually be assessed prior to kindergarten starting, unless they have been in a preschool special education program. The assessment may be the first time that some parents become aware that their children with SCA are showing any signs of difficulty with being academically "ready." Parents of children who had been receiving preschool special education may also be told that the level of disability is too small to continue to qualify for special services. Or a child may start in school, and the parents and teacher will realize that he or she is struggling. There are a variety of scenarios that will cause parents of children with SCA to convene the child study team (sometimes referred to as a Committee on Special Education, CSE, or other term) to evaluate or re-evaluate the child, and draw up an IEP.

Special education services for all school-age children are governed by the IEP, or individualized education program. It is a legal document backed by the IDEA legislation that details the therapy and educational services that will help the child to achieve developmental and educational milestones.

Parents actually have a great deal of power to initiate an evaluation or re-evaluation process to determine the exact services that must be delivered. By law, testing must be individualized and multi-disciplinary. Because parents of children with SCA may know more about the risks presented by their child's condition than school personnel, they can request a speech-language evaluation, OT and PT assessments, comprehensive neuropsychological testing, and a functional behavioral assessment (FBA), if necessary. A developmental pediatrician can help to justify the request to the school. If the testing seems cursory or inadequate, or the results of the testing seem inappropriate, the parent has the right to request, in writing, that the child be evaluated by a professional independent of the school district who specializes in the child's condition. The school district is obligated to pay for this independent testing.

> *From our experience, if I had not given the diagnosis of Trisomy X to the school, we would not have gotten any special education services, even with outside testing that we had done. The school said that our daughter was solidly average. The neuropsychological testing that we had performed privately told a completely different story of lots of deficits in learning and language that needed to be addressed.*
>
> *Having my son repeat kindergarten was probably the most helpful thing that we have done. In addition, we tried a number of multi-sensory programs, including the Orton-Gillingham reading method, resulting in his going from being way below grade reading level to being above-grade level. In addition, he does best in a small environment and by being pulled out of his classroom for reading and writing.*
>
> *In our opinion, push-in services have always been better for our daughter. We found that when she misses class, she falls further behind. When she is taught in an inclusion setting with the general education teacher and the special education teacher teaching side-by-side, she learns best.*
>
> *Our son's program has half special needs and half typically developing kids. He is typical in his cognitive and physical*

abilities, but he needs help with speech and language. If he were only in a special needs class, it would be to his detriment.

There are few professionals, outside of the EXtraordinarY Kids Clinic at the University of Colorado in Denver, who specialize in SCA, but many university-based developmental disabilities clinics have specialists in a number of disciplines who are familiar with SCA and can test appropriately for educational needs in a variety of cognitive and functional areas. If the parents decide to pay for testing and evaluation on their own, the special education team must also consider these testing results in drawing up an IEP.

Parents who are interested in learning more about their rights and responsibilities for helping to compose the IEP, as well how they can determine that the IEP is properly implemented, should familiarize themselves with www.wrightslaw.com, the leading special education and advocacy website in the U.S. It offers extensive information on the subject, as well as books and courses that parents will find invaluable as they navigate special education services for their children. It is far more useful to get information regarding special education regulations and practices from this website than for me to try to further digest it in this guide.

One guideline that I will give to parents who are contemplating initiating special education services, or to parents who already have them, is to communicate with the school in writing when making a request, and to follow up each meeting or conversation with a brief note thanking staff members for talking with you. State briefly what the results of the conversation were, and who holds responsibility for follow-up actions. If the results of the meeting are put into writing, it provides a record should there be later disputes that need resolution. Parents who write clear and respectful letters to their school districts almost automatically command respect and attention- because there is a record of all of the interactions.

It is also possible to address a child's learning needs without an IEP when the child is ineligible for special education services but has a disability requiring *accommodations* to help his learn effectively. This provision is **Section 504** of the Rehabilitation Act of 1973. The standard for a "504 Accommodation" is whether there is a physical or mental impairment, and whether the physical or mental impairment substantially limits one or more major life activities, including classroom performance. Basic modifications to teaching and testing can be done under a 504 plan, such as special placement in the classroom, additional time for testing, having instructions for assignments provided in writing, etc. Parents should realize, however, that a Section 504 plan does not have the legal weight of an IEP.

In order to fully provide for the child's needs in school, the parents may have to decide whether or not to disclose the diagnosis to the school. The downside of disclosure is that school personnel may go online, gain much misinformation, and then label the child based on old myths. The advantage of disclosing the diagnosis is that it provides the parent with the opportunity to educate school personnel accurately about SCA, and perhaps to obtain more individualized and effective services.

I found that I needed to speak individually to teachers to explain Klinefelter syndrome and its impact on John and his educational needs. School personnel were always receptive and grateful for the materials that I gave them. I did several in-service trainings at his schools, including speaking with all of the school nurses in special education facilities in our county on Long Island.

As students with extra X and Y chromosomes transition from elementary school into **middle school, junior high school, or high school**, the demands on them for work requiring greater written expression, for highly analytical work, and for much faster processing time, can cause a good student who previously needed no special services to begin to struggle. Parents need to be alert for signs that the academic demands on the student may require some accommodations under a 504 plan, or may require special services, such as reading lab, and an IEP. The process of requesting testing and a special education committee meeting is the same as described previously for preschool or elementary school.

Parents can provide some guidelines that can help teachers and other school staff to work more effectively with their children. A good understanding of your own child's strengths and weaknesses is the place that you can start. You can put this profile together from testing that has been done to justify either his IEP or his 504 plan. When speaking with school personnel or when working with the committee with which you create the IEP, provide a profile of your child with a bulleted listing of his characteristics. You may want to choose from some of the characteristics and strategies listed below to create a document that your child's teachers and other staff members can use for quick reference.

Strengths of children with extra X and Y chromosomes:

• Usually have much stronger receptive than expressive language: and will usually understand what is said and read to them

• Although they may have language-based learning disabilities, they are unlikely to have intellectual disability

• While it may take longer for a child with SCA to learn something, once the subject or task is learned, he or she will perform as well as any other student

• Non-verbal tasks including math, manual tasks such as art and gardening, computer skills and music are unlikely to be negatively impacted and are areas where the student may excel

• Children with SCA are usually more reserved and quiet than average in the classroom, and are not characterized by aggressive behavior, bullying, or risk-taking

• Children with SCA are usually quite curious and interested in quietly examining things in detail

• They like to please others and to be helpful

The student may experience challenges in the following areas:

• Short-term and working memory may be poor

• Executive functioning may be weak in the areas of 1) attention and ability to focus, 2) organization, 3) time management and activity planning, and 4) ability to transition between tasks and topics

• Language may be impaired, causing difficulty in verbal and written expression. Reading may also be made difficult and slowed by dyslexia and other specific disabilities

• Auditory processing may also be weak, making it more difficult for the student to follow directions and to remember material that is presented

• Fine motor skill deficits may make handwriting, coloring, artwork and other activities difficult and interfere with classroom performance

Strategies and interventions for addressing the learning needs of students with SCA:

• Children with SCA may require several repetitions of new information in order to learn the material, as well as visual cues (flash cards) and outlines to reinforce knowledge

• Reading and speech may be strengthened by teaching new vocabulary prior to reading material incorporating new words. Repetition is important in establishing knowledge of new vocabulary.

• Quiet and somewhat relaxed classroom environments are more productive with students who may be easily distracted. If necessary, the student should have the opportunity to work in a quiet corner of the classroom or in a reading lab, if necessary, if this is an effective means of allowing him or her to read or complete work

• Clear and predictable routines during the day help the student to transition from one activity to another

• Written instructions may be more effective than oral directions in allowing the student to understand assignments. Breaking down tasks into smaller steps will make the assignment easier for the student to understand and carry out

• Make certain that oral instructions and presentations are not provided too quickly. Children with SCA may need additional time to process information. They may be unable to write quickly enough to take good notes, and should be given the option of using a laptop computer, a recorder, or teacher's notes to help summarize material

• Students may be unable to organize their materials independently, and may require support to create and use a filing system, to learn to how to pack their backpacks, and to learn to use a daily planner.

• Older students may need specific instruction on study skills including:
1) how to take notes; 2) preparing for exams as well as reading and answering exam questions; 3) planning for, organizing and writing an essay; and 4) time management for studying

• For students who have fine motor skill challenges, teach keyboarding as early as possible, and investigate voice recognition technology to help older students compose written work on a computer

Behavioral and social challenges that may impact education:

• Children with SCA may have a tendency to withdraw from new people and new experiences

• They may be shy and appear to have difficulty fitting into the social network of a school. They may also miss social cues and have difficulty in making friends and in interacting with other students

• Because their language skills are often not equal to those of peers, they may appear quieter and less confident than other students

• Students with SCA may have difficulty in expressing emotions, and when frustrated by being unable to complete a task or understand directions, will demonstrate impulsive behavior, irritation, or a "meltdown"

• Students with SCA also experience anxiety at greater rates than their peers. They may suffer from lower self-esteem, particularly if they are bullied by other students

Some strategies that may be effective in addressing social and behavioral issues are:

• Involve the child in social skills training, including teaching "friendship" skills such as sharing, taking turns, and caring for others. If possible, use peer mentoring and match typically developing children with those with social skill deficits to model appropriate relation behavior

• Use the Social Stories method developed by Carol Gray to teach children to respond appropriately to social cues and to various situations at school

• Teach students self-advocacy skills and assertiveness techniques, and adopt a school-wide program to identify and stop bullying. Institute a school-wide program of celebrating inclusion of individuals with learning and other differences

• Teach the child to use positive language about himself and his wants and desires

• If the student is becoming frustrated, anxious, or angry, allow him to take a "time-out" and give him techniques to reduce tension. Some schools have time-out rooms for students with similar disabilities (autism, ADHD) who need to "chill out" until they can return to the classroom. Teach him anger management skills so that meltdowns are reduced.

If creating a 504 plan or an IEP for a child with SCA, it is also important to address some of the gross motor skill difficulties that he or she may experience. Physical education teachers need to know if a child has low muscle tone or lax and unstable joints, as well as poor coordination. Sometimes modifications in activities can be made so that the child can work more individually, if they desire, doing swimming, martial arts, golf, track, or another activity rather than competitive sports that require more coordination. If they are doing competitive sports, the physical education teacher may want to assign a position that will be easier for them to play successfully.

For adolescent boys with KS, it may be necessary to have a private talk with the school nurse and the physical education teacher in order to eliminate the need to shower with other students if the boy with KS is greatly behind in puberty or has gynecomastia that may be embarrassing when he is forced to undress in front of others.

For girls with Trisomy, Tetrasomy or Pentasomy X, dance and cheerleading are good activities when they are younger. Parents should be aware, however, that as steps and routines become more complicated, some girls will have difficulty following and remembering oral instructions, at the same time that poor coordination makes it more difficult for them to execute demanding maneuvers. Parents should voice their concerns about accommodations that may be necessary in physical education and make certain that this is written into the student's IEP or 504 plan.

Public school is not the only option when parents feel that their children are not being served appropriately, or when they prefer another setting. Private day and boarding school options exist that may provide smaller classes and better control over the student culture, so that children with SCA can learn and feel safe and nurtured. The cost of these options varies but it does present a barrier for many families. In limited cases, the public school district will pay for a private school placement. In other cases, and our family used this service, the school district will pay for services such as reading lab, speech therapy and social skills training, while the family pays for the basic private school tuition.

The best intervention was enrolling her in a private boarding high school for students with learning disabilities. It had small classes, lots of structure, and teachers who "got it." It was expensive but we used the money we had been saving for college when we realized that the path she was following would not lead to high school graduation unless we did something.

My son has been home schooled from the beginning because we felt that we could tailor his program exactly to his needs. Schools teach a certain amount of material within their 36-week time frame. We can stick with something longer if he is struggling. He isn't locked into one grade level. He can move ahead in subjects where he has no difficulty and spend long on subjects that are more difficult for him. It is a huge commitment and is not for everyone, but I feel that my son would not be where he is if he were in the standard educational system.

Another option to which a number of families with children with SCA have turned is homeschooling, often with the support of on-line resources, as well as small private schools that offer part-time enrichment and technical courses such as high school science and pre-college math. It should be possible to home-school a child and still obtain special education services from the district for which the child would have to travel to the school. If a child becomes overwhelmed with anxiety, and this certainly does happen with children with SCA, an active homeschooling program along with appropriate therapies can prevent him or her from falling behind. Homeschooling should be supplemented with group activities such as music, sports, and drama so that the student continues to have social interaction with other children on a regular basis. Check with your state for regulations covering homeschooling and to determine if documents must be filed with your school districts, and how assessments, if any, will be administered.

For high school students with SCA, planning for transition to post-secondary education (college, university, or technical school) or to the world of work and adulthood should begin by age fifteen. The chapter that follows covers "transition to adulthood," but there are important educational considerations that need to be addressed in the years prior to finishing high school. In the U.S., for special education students, planning should be discussed each annual meeting and documented in the I.E.P.

Education transition takes place when the young adult graduates from high school, which is usually at about age eighteen. Special education, students, however, have the right to remain in public school through age 21, although schools are reluctant to provide services to students for three additional years unless there are compelling learning or other disabilities to address. The decision about when to graduate from high school should depend on the student's academic progress as well as his maturity and ability to perform well in employment or in post-secondary education.

If a student requires very little accommodation to succeed academically, and he or she hasn't had to be "pushed" through school with a highly modified curriculum, then graduation at age eighteen makes sense, as long as there has been clear planning and preparation for work or education after graduation. If, however, the student is struggling academically, then parents should consider adding a vocational training and experience component to high school, even if this will add one or more years to high school.

Most public schools have available technical training programs and employment internships, often off-site and in settings more appropriate for young adults such as technical schools and community colleges. Graduation should not take place until the parent knows that the student can either succeed in a college program, or the student has gained enough employment skills and appropriate workplace behavior to obtain a job and be able to stay employed.

Once graduation takes place, the law that governs public school education in the U.S. for special education students, IDEA, no longer applies. IDEA mandates services for students requiring special education. After a student graduates and goes on to college or technical school, the law that governs education is the ADA, Americans with Disabilities Act of 1990.

I like math and was more successful with it than with reading and language. I graduated from high school but initially I could not make college work. I signed up for a class and attended until I knew I couldn't pass. I'd withdraw and take it again. By the third or fourth time, I could usually pass. Then I learned that I had dyslexia and needed extra help and accommodations. Once I got them, I was on the Dean's List. I secured my associates degree in Criminal Justice. Unfortunately, I couldn't become a police officer because the state would not allow me to have the qualifying exam read out loud to me and I couldn't pass it.

The school system, both high school and college, is simply not set up to accept and be helpful to people with learning disabilities. I had to fight with teachers regarding accommodations every year. The best advice I can give young adults is to find your voice early and not be afraid to speak up for your rights, otherwise the schools and colleges will "walk all over" you. This is good practice for when your parents can no longer speak on your behalf.

The ADA prohibits discrimination on the basis of disability, but it does not require that technical schools or colleges modify curriculum, provide alternate assessments, or make any other changes to guarantee that the student receives an education. Colleges and technical schools may make accommodations, such as providing class notes or a quiet place for taking exams and additional time for the exam, but they are not allowed to offer a different curriculum or to modify course requirements because of a student's disability. The student must self-identify as having a disability and must request assistance from the office providing services to students with disabilities. These offices often will not talk directly with the parent even if the student signs a form agreeing to let the disabilities services personnel communicate with his or her parent.

For students who have SCA, the transition to college or other postsecondary educational settings requires careful planning if there are learning disabilities and also if the student is somewhat immature, lacks strong executive functioning, or does not have well-developed social skills. The college workload requires that the student have the initiative to organize himself and to know when to ask for help. If the student has significant learning disabilities, you may want to locate a college with a very strong learning services program, which may be available at extra cost. *Peterson's* and *Princeton Review* are among the excellent guides to colleges with specific support programs. For students who have difficulty with standardized testing, many colleges do not require either the ACT or the SAT test.

Although "going away" to college is a goal for many, the student should consider whether he can manage both the workload as well as negotiate the social life and the demands of living away from home in a dorm setting. For many students, starting out their college careers in a community college as a commuter allows them to adjust first to the academic rigors of college, without having to also manage life independently in a dorm. By the time that students have completed two years of college, they are far better prepared for a larger campus as well as for life on-campus or in an apartment.

Transitioning from School to Adulthood

The process of attaining adulthood and the beginnings of independence from family is referred to as "transition to adulthood," or often, just "transition." For young people with any special health care needs or developmental issues, transition can provide an additional challenge beyond the typical difficulties of learning to coordinate it all: finances, decision-making, lifestyle choices, career, and relationships.

Young adults with extra X and Y chromosomes may be less mature than their peers, which can add to the stress of taking on new responsibilities on graduation from high school. If, in addition, the young person also has difficulty with anxiety, or executive functioning, or learning disabilities, then transitioning to adulthood and to independence may require more support, and for a longer period, than for siblings and peers.

For parents, it is often a bit difficult to tell how transition will progress, and what barriers there may be to achieving independence. It is important to begin to understand the process of transition well ahead of the child's eighteenth birthday, which is considered the point at which he or she becomes an adult. Parents should also become familiar with the issues that their children will face on reaching adulthood, and begin to plan four to five years before this actually occurs.

I want him to be able to fulfill some of his dreams, live on his own and be a productive person. I want him to have healthy relationships and to be a happy person. I do worry about future bullying and how mean and harsh people can be with others who are different.

I seems that most people with SCA that I meet or find online go through the same general cycle of being a "late bloomer." It would be nice to warn parents of what will come—eventual success as an adult—and perhaps even create a class for parents taught by those of us who have the condition.

The range of functioning of adolescents with SCA makes planning for transition difficult for parents. Because the expression of these genetic conditions is so broad, one may have to plan for both a child whose progress into adulthood is relatively routine and successful as well as for the child who may remain financially and emotionally dependent on family and government benefits temporarily or even throughout his or her lifetime. The emphasis of this section covering transition to adulthood is that families of children with SCA need to plan for and support the adolescent in maximizing achievement and progress toward independence, while preserving their rights to government benefits and other vocational and life skills supports that may become necessary.

My husband and I always believed that because John did reasonably well academically in a high school environment, he would certainly succeed at least in earning an associate's degree, and in obtaining paid employment by the age of 21 or 22. John was not able to accomplish either a two-year degree or successful and continuous employment, although he certainly tried. His executive functioning turned out to be too weak and his learning disabilities too significant for him to achieve this without far more support than we had planned he would need.

Although we thought it might be possible that he would require some level of vocational assistance, we did not set out to qualify him for government benefits (Supplemental Security Income, or SSI) or for services from New York State's Office for Persons with Developmental Disabilities. Our belief was that if he thought he could receive SSI funds without having to work, he would not apply himself toward getting a job. We also thought that he probably functioned at too high a level to qualify for services for those with developmental disabilities. Fortunately, however, we had been advised when he was in high school to place any financial assets for him in a Supplemental Needs

Trust, just in case he should need government benefits. Following through on this advice meant that we were prepared when it became clear that he would need a significant level of government support to begin to live independently.

We did apply for SSI for John when he was 21 and it was granted along with Medicaid. We had also applied for services through New York State's offices for vocational rehabilitation and for persons with developmental disabilities. John received job coaching and assistance with finding a job immediately. It took several years of waiting before he was granted life skills training and other services through the developmental disabilities agency.

We moved him into an apartment living program for high-functioning young people who require assistance with achieving independence, supplementing his rent out-of-pocket because he is considered to be too "high-functioning" to qualify for housing assistance. He does have some social life now, as well as a good relationship with his life-skills trainer who is teaching him how to live independent of us. At the time that this guide was written, he was 23, and living independently in the community fairly successfully. Before we obtained government benefits for him, however, we could not see how he would build a satisfying life.

Some of the major elements of transition include:

- Legal status change from child to adult
- Educational programming
- Vocational training and employment
- Medical services and decision-making
- Life skills (personal care, money management, nutrition, housekeeping)
- Financial support
- Residential arrangements
- Family relationships

The most significant change on reaching age eighteen is that the child's legal status changes from that of a dependent to that of a competent adult. The law assumes that an adult is responsible for medical and financial decision-making. Unless various legal documents are filed, including such instruments as "**power of attorney**," full or partial "**guardianship**," or an "**authorization to communicate protected health information**," parents may find that they no longer have any right to assist their adult children with these decisions, even if the young adult is not ready to take responsibility for such actions independently.

As children approach age eighteen, parents need to ask themselves if their sons or daughters are going to be able to function independently with these responsibilities, at least initially. Do they understand their medical care needs sufficiently to be able to interact independently with their health care providers, or do they require assistance to choose among therapies, schedule appointments, and refill prescriptions? Is the young person capable of understanding and signing a contract to open a credit card account, or to purchase a car with a car loan? Can he understand the basics of tax regulations and appropriately income file tax returns?

If the answer to any of these questions "no," then the parent needs to determine how it is most appropriate to proceed with completing some legal documentation that will permit the parent to continue to assist with decision-making and to be recognized as a legal agent of the adult son or daughter.

Because these are legal instruments, every state and country has its own provisions to allow one person to make decisions for another. In general, there is law allowing people without any developmental disability or mental illness to grant decision-making rights. There is also separate law that grants decision-making to parents or other responsible parties when the person has a developmental disability or other illness that renders the person unable to make such decisions. Parents will need to research the provisions that cover their adult child in their state or country of residence.

The easiest provision to put in effect, in the United States, is "durable power of attorney" in which the adult grants his parents decision-making authority for medical, financial, and other decisions. Most countries have similar instruments. The adult must be competent to understand what he is signing which means that he or she must not have severe or profound intellectual disability, dementia, or mental illness. The adult also has the right to revoke all or some of the provisions that he or she granted at any time, for any reason.

For the majority of young adults with SCA, who have decent relations with their parents, and who may need and want assistance with such matters as banking, taxes, and medical care, power of attorney is an inexpensive and appropriate measure for providing assistance until the young adult is ready to take on such matters independently. Spouses often sign these documents, which can also serve as instruments for making end-of-life decisions, if that ever were necessary.

In the United State, HIPAA (Health Care Portability and Accountability Act) provides for strong protection measures for health care communication and information. It is the law that if a young adult bars his physician from communicating with his parents, the physician cannot legally do so, unless there is a life-threatening situation. Many health care providers protect themselves by requiring that any patient sign an authorization telling them with whom they may legally communicate. The parent should take the opportunity when his child turns eighteen to complete these forms so that there will be no question of the ability to communicate about health care issues.

Guardianship generally applies only where there is significant developmental disability or mental illness present. The majority of families with adult children with SCA will not want to or need to petition for guardianship. It is often appropriate in cases of intellectual disability, when there is severe and persistent mental illness such as bipolar disorder or schizophrenia, or when the person with SCA also has an autism spectrum disorder. Guardianship requires documentation from one or more physicians that the person is unable to understand or make reasonable medical and financial decisions due to the illness or developmental disability. The guardianship is often only granted by a judge after a hearing. It may be contested by the individual. Generally, guardianship is permanent and requires appointing back-up guardians such as siblings or other relatives.

Employment is often the standard by which success as a young adult is measured, whether immediately following high school or after graduation from college or vocational training. The results of our survey told us that getting established in a career, whether after high school or after vocational training or college, could be problematic for the young adults with SCA.

Workplace skills often are quite different from what makes someone a good student, so that even those young people who had quite a strong academic performance could find employment challenging. One of the reasons for this is that entry level jobs often require exceptionally good social skills, and the ability to "get along" with co-workers and with the public. If someone is a bit withdrawn or shy, they may be seen as not being a team player. This is further complicated if the employee has difficulty in understanding instructions that are given verbally and quickly, or if the employee is left on his own to "figure it out," and this makes him or her anxious, further limiting the ability to perform.

What we found from the survey is that finding the right "fit" in employment can be a trial and error process. Young adults with SCA do not look any different from the norm, and if they have learning disabilities, they are often mild to moderate in severity. Motor skill deficits, if present, are subtle and not obvious at first glance. They have intelligence in the normal range, and for this reason, are often not referred for vocational services during or after high school. The combination of small deficits, however, in verbal skills, auditory processing of information, strength and dexterity, sequencing and prioritization of tasks, however, can add up to overall difficulty in performing on the job and in retaining employment.

I worry about my future constantly. I worry that I won't do well in college or that I will have to drop out and then never be able to get a good paying job. My social anxiety keeps me as an 19-year-old from being able to get a job and from learning to drive. I still do not even have a learner's permit.

My son has not matured as much as his peers. He prefers to be alone and has not had many friends since grade school. His social skills are way behind his age. He does well with older adults but he is not comfortable with his peers. I fear that his struggles with social skills will be what keeps him from getting and keeping a job.

If a young adult with SCA is having difficulty with either finding a job initially or with staying employed, there are numerous resources to which he or she can turn. All states have vocational rehabilitation services that can provide assistance to people who have a disability that presents a barrier to employment. The key seems to be to obtain help before a pattern of unemployment sets in, along with the depression and avoidance that can result from losing one job after another. One resource for locating vocational rehabilitation services is www.ilru.org, which provides addresses and websites of Independent Living Centers in the U.S. as well as internationally. All such centers can refer you to vocational rehabilitation resources.

Agencies that provide employment services require medical evidence of disability, which means revealing the diagnosis of SCA to the rehabilitation counselor. The counselor may know nothing about SCA, so it is important for the family and the young adult to educate the counselor. Emphasize the combination of subtle disabilities that often characterize the workplace performance of the person with SCA. The services that are provided by vocational rehabilitation services are usually free, and can include psychological testing, vocational aptitude assessments, training programs, job placement assistance and job coaching, or support once the client has found employment.

Often, the state does not actually provide the service but contracts it out to non-profit agencies and other vendors. When looking for an appropriate agency for vocational services, persons with SCA often do well in settings that are accustomed to working with the population of persons with high-functioning autism or Asperger syndrome, or with persons with other neurological impairments. If you can locate an agency that specializes in placing and supporting clients who do not have intellectual disability, the employment identified may require a higher skill level, even though it will often be "entry" level, in data processing, cashiering, customer service, manufacturing, etc.

Once on the job, the employee may discover that there are accommodations that need to be made so that he or she can be successful. For those who continue to have low muscle tone, standing all day at a cash register or computer may prove to be impossible. Having a stool to sit on would be considered a reasonable accommodation. If the employee has difficulty with taking in and remembering multi-part verbal instructions, having instructions for the day put in writing is also a reasonable accommodation. This does require disclosing the disability to the employer, but it also provides some protection under ADA for the employee. For employees who need advice on appropriate requests for accommodations on the job, the Independent Living Centers referenced previously provide assistance as can agencies that provide vocational programs.

Medical transition to adult care is another area to manage. By the age of eighteen, children with SCA should have been given as much information about their genetic conditions as possible. Children who have been getting their care from a pediatrician need to transition to an adult physician by the time that they are eighteen to twenty-one. For any young adults who have been receiving specialty care, such as endocrinology, from a pediatric specialist, a transfer will also need to be made to an adult specialist.

Although young adults will often want to continue to have their parents involved in medical visits, they will need to sign appropriate forms to continue to have the health care providers communicate with their parents. This is a good opportunity to begin to transfer responsibility for making appointments and for refilling prescriptions to the young adult.

When locating an adult physician, ask your child's pediatric health care providers for practitioners who are likely to be familiar with or open to learning about SCA, and any possible health care implications for adulthood. You may need to interview physicians, and to ask them if they are familiar with the diagnosis. Bring some literature with you, and observe how they respond to being given written material or to having you tell them about the conditions. The decision regarding a new provider has to be shared by the young adult.

Medical insurance coverage is another area of concern, particularly in the U.S. Previously, SCA was considered to be a risk factor that could make obtaining insurance outside of employer plans difficult. It could be excluded as a "pre-existing condition" or the cost of the insurance could be increased to cover real or speculative risks of complications. After the health care reforms of 2010, children can no longer be excluded from policies due to pre-existing conditions. In addition, young adults, who would normally be dropped from their parents' policies on leaving high school or college, can now continue to be covered until age 26. Those who are over 26 and do not have insurance coverage through an employer may need to wait until 2014 to be guaranteed coverage through insurance pools and through subsidies. Some states have low-cost insurance for low income persons. There is also the option of Medicaid for young adults covered by SSI, or for young adults who meet income and disability qualifications for it.

Prescription drug coverage is another concern, particularly for those who require hormone replacement and other maintenance drug therapy for conditions such as ADHD, high cholesterol or diabetes. Most drug companies have patient assistance programs that will provide the drugs at no cost or very low cost ($10–$15 per month) provided that income limitations are met. Information for these programs is available on-line at the websites of the pharmaceutical company that manufactures the required drug.

Financial considerations in adulthood include how much support a young person may need to attend college or to become established in a job as well as to move out into an apartment. Whether or not a family provides financial assistance to the young adult is an individual decision and depends on the family's resources as well as the young adult's ability to work and to earn a living wage.

There are several important additional considerations when a young adult has SCA. For many, SCA does not necessarily mean developmental disability, but it can mean developmental delay. That delay can be in developing the maturity to train for a career, and to be able to work full-time and become self-supporting. Or, the young adult may truly qualify as having a developmental disability because of having a seizure disorder, meeting the criteria for an autism spectrum disorder, or having borderline intelligence or true intellectual disability. Some adults also develop complications after school ends, such as autoimmune disorders or serious mental illness, that makes them incapable of becoming self-supporting.

If an adult child is not able to support him or herself, even temporarily, parents have several options. These include providing financial assistance outright and applying for government disability benefits. In the US, these benefits are provided by the Federal Government and are administered by the Social Security Administration for persons with disabilities that limit their ability to earn income. It is a good idea to have thought about this possibility prior to a child's graduation from high school, and to discuss it with your spouse or partner so that there is agreement on how to approach financial assistance if it becomes necessary, or if you know that the young adult is likely to require support.

If parents choose to provide financial support, they should make this contingent on the young adult's making adequate and measurable progress toward independence. This may mean setting, perhaps with the assistance of a counselor, realistic goals for attending training programs, looking for work, participating in counseling or therapy, taking medication, and performing chores around the house that contribute to the household. A written contract for assistance is not a bad idea. If parents provide a car and insurance, that is also part of financial support, and there should be a contract for what the parents expect in return. Open-ended financial assistance does not provide the young adult with any incentive to become self-supporting. Parents should avoid this trap by setting terms for the support, and clear consequences when the adult son or daughter fails to uphold his or her end of the contract.

> *His lack of impulse control can get him into trouble, especially with money. I hope that he will be able to manage his finances as he has a tendency to spend every dollar that gets.*
>
> *She will never be financially self-sufficient. She doesn't have the capability of living completely on her own. We are working toward independence, and will assist her in getting a condominium. I have started a "Registered Disability Savings Plan" for her. It will allow me to set up a trust fund to supplement whatever she earns or receives in social assistance. I hope that her brother or sister will help to oversee this, but it is a lot to ask.*

When providing financial support, it is also useful to take measures to make certain that young adults understand financial responsibility before providing them too much latitude with things like credit cards. All young people, regardless of any disability, need to start out money management with a debit card that limits over-expenditures, rather than a credit card with a high credit limit. If he or she has a cell phone, a car, or internet or cable service, provide a set allowance to the young person, and have the young person pay for these expenses out of the allowance. Provide opportunities to learn about finances by having the young adult take responsibility for living within a reasonable budget, and resist the temptation to provide loans to bail out an adult child who overspends or uses funds too quickly in a month. If necessary, provide weekly allowance until the young person learns to budget successfully to make funds last for two or more weeks.

Another option, which can be in addition to family financial support, is to apply for **Supplemental Security Income** (SSI) after the child turns eighteen if the inability to earn enough money to be self-supporting is due to disability. SSI is administered by the Social Security Administration and provides income support for persons who, *because of a disability*, are unable to engage in *substantial gainful employment*, which is defined to mean, in 2011, the inability to work in competitive employment and earn at least $1000 per month. (In some cases, the individual will be eligible for Social Security Disability Income because of a parent's retirement or disability. This will be determined by the Social Security Administration when application is made, and does not change the application process or the criteria for determining eligibility.)

The reason for applying after eighteen is that when a child turns eighteen, he will have only his own financial assets and income considered in the application, not the income or assets of the parent. In order to qualify, the applicant must have assets of less than $2000 *in his own name*, and he may not earn more than $1000 per month.

If a parent believes that there is a reasonable chance that he will need to apply for SSI for an adult child at age eighteen, or within several years of the eighteenth birthday, the parent should take action before the child turns fifteen or sixteen to move any assets out of the child's name and into a **supplemental needs trust.** These trusts are designed specifically for persons with disabilities and other medical conditions that may require them to access government benefits such as SSI and Medicaid to pay for services such as medical care, income support, supportive or therapeutic housing, and life skills training. The trusts allow the funds to be used for all purposes except housing, food and clothing, while maintaining eligibility for the person with special needs for government benefits. Such trusts must be established by attorneys or agencies with expertise in special needs benefit law and estate planning.

The laws governing these trusts in the U.S. are both Federal and state, and vary by location.

If you do apply for SSI, the process is described in detail in an excellent website: www.ssa.gov. In order to qualify, the applicant must have a disabling condition that causes his or her inability to earn at least $1000 per month, and there must be adequate medical documentation to demonstrate this. Sex chromosome aneuploidy (SCA), by itself, is not considered to be a "listed" medical condition that will automatically qualify a person for disability as determined by SSI. There must be additional co-morbid medical and psychiatric conditions present, and there must be strong medical documentation provided by physicians and psychologists confirming this. If the medical documentation is weak, the applicant will have to see an SSI physician, and these physicians are unlikely to be helpful to someone with SCA in documenting disability.

The application can be opened by phone, using the 800 number on the website, and the documentation can be completed on-line, which is a process that may take three or more hours. An applicant with a learning disability should obtain help in completing the application. It may also be helpful to have an advocate or attorney specializing in Social Security prepare the application and represent the applicant before Social Security. The cost of these advocates is reasonable and can greatly reduce the rate of denial, which is substantial because many disability examiners are unfamiliar with SCA.

Once SSI has been granted, applicants are allowed to work and to earn up to $1400 per month, with benefits reduced by approximately $1 for every $2 earned. In most states, qualifying for SSI will automatically also qualify the recipient for Medicaid, which can pay for medical bills, prescriptions, and other supportive services for persons with developmental disability or psychiatric conditions. Persons with SCA are not considered permanently disabled, and will be evaluated periodically to determine that they still meet the criteria for coverage. Coverage by SSI or SSDI, however, can buy additional time for a young person who is having difficulty becoming established in employment to gain skills and become self-supporting.

Life skills include the behaviors that young adults must develop in order to gain independence successfully. Money management, discussed previously, is one such life skill. So are self-care, appropriate grooming, hygiene, nutrition, exercise, and health maintenance. Housekeeping skills, including cleaning, laundry, food shopping and preparation, and simple home maintenance are critical life skills. Safety considerations include food safety and knowledge of avoidance of toxins, fire prevention and detection, locking doors and home security measures, internet and phone security, guarding of personal identity, and travel safety and appropriate use of alcohol. Young adults also need an understanding of basic principles of law, as well as knowing their legal rights should they have contact with law enforcement.

> *I think that my biggest revelation was that I had to come to terms with her capabilities and balance them against her safety. It was tough. When she came of drinking age she loved going out to loud clubs and drinking and dancing and then putting up all sorts of inappropriate photos on her Facebook page. Her sister finally got through to her so that she now recognizes an inappropriate photo and puts only appropriate material on Facebook*

Most adolescents and young adults learn life skills in the course of growing up from observing their family members and from their peers. If there are learning disabilities or developmental delays, assimilation of life skills may be incomplete. The problem is that life skills are generally specifically taught as a curriculum only to relatively low-functioning young people with intellectual disability in school, or in centers for those with significant developmental disabilities. For most of the population of those with SCA, there will be few opportunities available to learn life skills unless parents identify their children's deficits and take measures to remedy this.

Some young adults with SCA may be eligible for public services for those with developmental or psychiatric disabilities. Eligibility varies significantly by state and by country. Particularly if a young adult has a 48- or 49-chromosome variation of SCA, or also has a co-morbid diagnosis of autism spectrum, seizure, psychiatric, or other neurological disorder, he or she may be eligible for these services. Life skills instruction is often provided by life skills trainers who come into the home. Public programs may be associated with supportive apartment programs that provide part-time life skills training services. Eligibility usually requires that the young adult also be receiving SSI or SSDI and be covered by Medicaid.

There are also private post-secondary programs designed for high-functioning young people who need life skills instruction to learn to live independently. Sometimes these programs are combined with vocational preparation and community college training, such as the College Living Experience (www.experiencecle.com), the Vocational Independence Program, Riverview School GROW Program, Minnesota Life College, and others. They are usually residential programs, and are relatively expensive, but they provide a good grounding in life skills and usually lead to the opportunity to work and live in an apartment. Some programs offer continuing residential services for young adults living in apartments that involve part-time life skills training as well as vocational coaching and some social programming. A variety of public and private funds can support adults who take part in these programs. My son is part of such an apartment program that operates in metropolitan New York.

An on-line resource for parents and others who want to create an individual training program for a person with SCA is the Casey Life Skills curriculum. Originally created by the Annie E. Casey Foundation to teach adolescents in foster care the skills that they would need to live independently as adults, the online site, http://www.caseylifeskills.org/index.htm, offers an assessment, a curriculum, and teaching activities that are appropriate for high-functioning young adults with SCA who need to learn basic living skills.

As adolescents become adults and begin separating from family, their **relationships with family and parents** change. For parents of sons and daughters who may have had significant learning and developmental challenges and delays, it may take concerted effort to begin "letting go" as the young person enters adulthood. All young adults need to begin taking on increasing responsibility as they are able to manage particular areas of their lives. They also need to have the opportunity to make mistakes, to fail in certain areas and to learn from these mistakes. It is difficult for a parent who has had to advocate constantly for a child to begin to step back and coach him or her to do so independently. This is particularly true for a parent whose child with SCA has reached young adulthood, and still requires some support in specific areas.

As a parent whose 23-year-old son still gets some financial support from home, and who requires life skills coaching to live independently, I know that stepping back is difficult. It is also sometimes the case that when I tell John that he is responsible for taking on certain tasks, like making his own doctor appointments and refilling his own prescriptions, he indicates that he would rather I continue to do it for him. Although it might be easier to continue to do these functions myself, I make a point of transferring them to John to do with help from his life skills trainer.

Once a young person attains adulthood, parents need to constantly assess what they do for their adult son or daughters. If it is an area where the young adult can assume responsibility without substantial risk of financial or other harm, then provide advice and coaching from a distance, but otherwise transfer the responsibility. Failure to step back and allow young adults to make mistakes -unless the mistakes or failure would be clearly damaging- risks fostering too much dependence in their adult children. It also is most likely to result in building resentment on the part of their adult children, who feel that their parents are retaining too much control.

All of this is a balancing act for parents of young adults with special needs, and there is nothing easy about it.

From the small number of research studies that have followed people with SCA into adulthood, and from our survey completed for purposes of informing this guide, we do know that the large majority of individuals with SCA do attain independence in adulthood. They describe their adult lives as satisfying, although they acknowledge the barriers that they faced as adolescents and young adults. Their parents, not surprisingly, continue to express concerns, even when the young adults have moved out into their own homes, established careers and developed adult relationships which may include marriage and children. The same can be said for parents of typically developing children who have grown up, although the extent of concern is not usually so great.

What's Next?

There is little as self-indulgent as writing and self-publishing the book that one has always wanted to have available, in this case a fairly comprehensive guide to X and Y chromosome variations. I dreamed of being able to research and write this guide for several years before the opportunity of retiring early at age 59 presented itself in 2010. In fact, I took on the project of interviewing individuals with these chromosomal conditions as well as parents and other relatives over the year before I started writing. I also created an online survey using www.surveymonkey.com that I expected would attract perhaps 200 participants to tell me about their lives or their family members; I received more than 800 responses. Those responses shaped the materials presented in the guide.

It is clear to me, however, that the state of knowledge regarding X and Y chromosome variations is still quite limited despite a slowly increasing volume of research into and publications addressing Klinefelter syndrome, Trisomy X, 47,XYY and their 48 and 49 chromosome variants. Awareness of the genetic conditions is low, among both the general public as well as professionals, particularly among those in health care who are in a position to both suspect the diagnosis and order testing that would confirm the presence of the genetic condition. This last short section is a further indulgence for me, providing me an opportunity to present my "wish list" for improving the lives of those with X and Y chromosome variations, as well as their family members and loved ones.

Although **"awareness" campaigns** have probably been overdone in this country, what the X and Y chromosome variations community needs is an awareness campaign. In my early career, I worked in the pulmonary program at the University of Michigan and we promoted early detection and diagnosis of cystic fibrosis with the slogan, "Kiss your baby" so that parents who detected a salty taste would bring it to their pediatrician's attention. It probably is true that the public, and parents in particular, will influence early detection if they know the constellation of symptoms that are indications for genetic testing.

Capturing public attention can be a challenge because while featuring a genetic condition in the popular media can jumpstart the process, it isn't easy to be picked up by the most influential sources, including popular television shows such as *Dr. Oz* or the Sunday *New York Times Magazine.* SCA is a hidden disability, much like Asperger syndrome and high-functioning autism were fifteen years ago. The additional barrier is that many individuals and parents are reluctant to disclose the diagnosis, because of its inaccurate association with criminal behavior, so finding celebrities and other public figures willing to use their names to help publicize the condition is not as likely as with other medical conditions.

At the same time as public awareness of these relatively common disorders is built, the SCA community has to create easily **accessible, authoritative and comprehensive web-based information** for persons who receive such a diagnosis or need accurate information about it. KS&A is beginning to bring its website up to this level of sophistication, particularly with the advent of its "webinars," but it also needs to have available concise downloadable brochures that summarize the individual conditions, as well as bibliographies and links to the best of the publically accessible scientific literature.

In addition, KS&A and other major support organizations for individuals with SCA need the funding to build the **infrastructure of national or international support organizations**. The infrastructure should provide for public relations, support services for the newly diagnosed, family and professional education programs, and promotion of research initiatives. My position is that the pharmaceutical manufacturers who market hormone preparations as well as the psychotropic medications on which this population relies bear some responsibility for providing resources to the SCA community, but so far this hasn't occurred. Clearly, building such a support organization requires an effective fundraising campaign that pulls in a variety of interests beyond individuals and families. We might try to work with organizations that focus on disability rights as well as finding common ground with organizations that seek to reduce the rate of fetal abortion.

The rate of publication about X and Y chromosome variations in medical and other professional journals has increased substantially in the past decade. It is time, however, for development and publication of an **authoritative textbook** covering the conditions. When a set of conditions has a textbook devoted to their diagnosis and treatment, health care professionals are more likely to consult that text when researching treatment for particular patients. More important, health care trainees will have in one volume comprehensive and detailed information that they can access and will remember once they are in practice. It is my goal to work with a number of the professionals that have made SCA a focus of their practice to help coordinate such a text with multiple authors.

At the same time, the SCA community needs to be promoting development of **care plans and treatment standards** for both pediatric and adult populations. Care plans consist of indications for diagnosis as well as diagnostic standards, and establish a standard of care and care protocols for these conditions. They are developed by professional working groups and adopted by organizations such as the American Academy of Pediatrics.

Organizations that serve the SCA population have always said that a major goal is to have accurate training about SCA incorporated into **medical school curriculum**, so that X and Y chromosome variations are considered when undertaking differential diagnosis of developmental and learning disabilities, or particular constellations of symptoms, such as low muscle tone, delayed puberty, and tremors. It is also a goal to have available more detailed training for genetic counselors, psychologists, speech therapists, and others who work with this population. In addition to training for the young doctors and other health care and education professionals, a series of web-based as well as conventional lecture-based **continuing education programs** need to be developed for primary care physicians, specialists, and other health professionals. If we are going to promote early diagnosis by publicizing the condition to families and individuals, then we need to also have trained personnel ready to offer the standard of care for X and Y chromosome variations.

One of the single most effective developments in meeting these goals has been the establishment of the EXtraordinarY Kids Clinic at the University of Colorado Children's Hospital by Dr. Nicole Tartaglia and her associates. Finally, families facing a diagnosis of SCA have a clinic that offers "one-stop shopping." This multi-specialty clinic addresses the many clinical and educational manifestations that may present in X and Y chromosome variations. Not only is the clinic the leader in establishing clinical guidelines for managing SCA, it also serves as a model for clinical training as well as specialized research into these disorders. The problem, obviously, is that it is one clinic serving the population of the U.S. as well as the rest of the world. The wait to get an appointment is long, even though most families must travel a significant distance at considerable expense. Clearly, another item on the agenda is to **establish additional clinics** devoted to X and Y chromosome variations in the United States at major academic medical centers, as well as clinics in other countries around the world. Once this begins to occur, it will indicate that tertiary medical centers now view this relatively common set of disorders as clinically valuable to providing comprehensive medical care. Training programs will be strengthened, and clinical and translational research initiatives addressing SCA will expand.

There are many disorders that have been viewed in the past as associated with "shame," and sex chromosome aneuploidy is certainly high up on that list. Not only is the term, "sex," associated with the conditions, thus making the diagnosis questionable in the eyes of rather prudish Americans, but there are the old myths of predisposition to criminality with which the population has to contend. On top of that,

Klinefelter syndrome is associated with infertility and therefore with being unable to function fully as a male. In addition, there is certainly a significant minority of those with 47,XXY, who have gender identity issues or who are openly gay or bisexual.

I don't believe that the SCA community can make substantial progress toward the goal of having these diagnoses seen as medical and developmental conditions until they are able to erase the stigma associated with X and Y chromosome variations. To some extent, it is a "chicken or egg" problem: Because of the potential stigma, we avoid disclosing the diagnosis outside of the immediate family, and we might use alternative labels, such as Asperger syndrome or ADHD, to describe our loved ones to schools or to friends. Giving a more acceptable label, of course, means that fewer lay people and professionals have the opportunity to learn about SCA and its constellation of possible symptoms, so it continues to be thought of as a rare disorder. And reluctance to disclose the diagnosis perpetuates the stigma, both for the individual and the family, and for the general public.

And with respect specifically to the gender identity and sexual preference **diversity** of the 47,XXY, population, the SCA community has to acknowledge this as one manifestation of the genetic phenotype. For many people, particularly those with conservative religious and social views, it may be a real challenge to embrace this as a consequence of genetic and hormonal variation. I am understanding of those who may view this from a different set of moral standards, but the evidence is increasingly strong that people who are gay and bisexual, or who have gender dysphoria or see themselves as intersex, do not choose this dilemma for themselves. They are born with these differences, and there is increasing evidence that genetics plays a strong role. To the extent that those of us who want X and Y chromosome variations to be seen strictly as medical and developmental conditions, it isn't possible to be accepting most of the phenotypic manifestations, while continuing to believe that the sexual orientation and gender identity issues are stigmatizing, and therefore better kept secret.

The final goal in my wish list is that there be far more research into these genetic conditions throughout the lifespan as well as into treatment for the various symptoms. This is potentially a very valuable population to study because we know what the extra chromosome is, and where there may or may not be extra genetic "dosing," making it potentially a model for studying brain development or predisposition to various disorders, such as autoimmune disease or autism. Adults with extra X and Y chromosomes have relatively little information about how the conditions may affect aging, and many of the adults responding to the survey spoke of their concerns about the chromosomal condition's impact on their health as they grow older. At some point in the future, I would hope that the advocacy organizations such as KS&A can raise sufficient funds to provide seed money grants to researchers so that they can go on to make application for major funding through government agencies, such as the National Institutes of Health.

I don't know how long it will take to achieve these goals for X and Y chromosome variations. KS&A did set the research initiative moving with several scientific conferences that it funded and ran in the mid-1990s. The researchers then went on to organize their own international conferences in 2009 and 2010. There is every indication that this research direction will continue as more scientists become interested in the myriad of clinical questions to explore.

Until I had finished this guide, I chose not to be on the Board of KS&A, even though it would have allowed me to influence some of the organization's activities. I was reluctant to join the Board because until several years ago, there was significant pressure on participants in the organization not to disclose the full extent of medical and developmental complications that can affect children and adults who have SCA. We were discouraged from exploring the tie between autism spectrum disorders and SCA, or even mentioning an SCA diagnosis in the same sentence as "developmental disability." And certainly, no one was to discuss whether homosexuality might possibility occur at a higher rate among men who are 47,XXY, than among men who are 46,XY. In order to retain my independence, this guide was published completely independently. Once having accomplished that, however, I then decided that I would be open to accepting a Board membership if it were offered, and I was nominated and elected.

I would hope that the majority of my wish list can be accomplished in the next ten years. That would mean that no more families and individuals would find themselves facing a new and scary diagnosis with little guidance from health care professionals, and with access only to cursory and generalized information, unless they were in a position to access medical literature. Their own primary care physicians would have basic knowledge about SCA and would be able to make referrals to specialty clinics within a reasonable distance for consultation and treatment recommendations.

Accomplishing the goals on my wish list would also mean that a much higher percentage of children who have developmental and learning difficulties would benefit from early diagnosis, because SCA would be on the "radar" of pediatricians and special educators, and part of careful differential diagnosis, instead of frequently being discovered only by accident, and often late in a child's development, or in adulthood. The conditions would be recognized as making children eligible for early intervention and for special education services, if necessary. Vocational placement agencies would recognize the potential challenges of working with young adults with SCA, and would understand workplace accommodations that could help them to achieve success on the job.

Perhaps more important that anything else, the stigma surrounding a diagnosis of sex chromosome aneuploidy would disappear. Genetic counselors and obstetricians would not feel an obligation to warn parents against ever disclosing the diagnosis. And as children become adolescents and adults, they will not feel that they have a genetic condition, something so integral to their sense of self, which they need to hide. This is downplayed, in my estimation, as a factor in the very low self-esteem of many adolescents and adults who have extra X and Y chromosomes. I think that it is critical that the SCA community take effective action to change this. X and Y chromosome variations can then be seen as the fascinating genetic, endocrine, and developmental conditions that they are, and treated accordingly.

Acknowledgments

I am truly fortunate to have fallen into the opportunity to write this book, and to have had the support of numerous friends and colleagues, and my own family, that made this possible. Retirement is a wonderful thing, but I am very glad that I was able to throw myself into this project, rather than wasting time with puttering around the house, and finally cleaning out the closets. Producing a guide for families and individuals to this common, and yet largely unknown medical and developmental condition, is far more satisfying than a clean closet.

There is no "market" for such a book, at least as recognized by the major publishers, so I relied on many people with whom I have become acquainted during this journey to learn about and make sense of sex chromosome aneuploidy. In fact, many of my long-time friendships have grown through the various support groups and organizations that provide information and advocacy for this population. KS&A, while not directly involved with the development and content of this guide, provided internet publicity for the online survey that provided so much information for the book. Other organizations and list-serves, most of them virtual, provided assistance in gathering the data.

Amy Turiff provided her expertise as a genetic counselor and as a researcher in this field, helping me with the composition of the survey and its analysis, as well as reading the text and helping me to portray the genetics of SCA in a clear and accurate, yet understandable manner for laypersons. Jim Moore of KS&A, along with Sandra Henson, Gary Glissman, Myra Byrd, and numerous other members (some preferring anonymity) read the materials and provided invaluable comments. Dr. Nicole Tartaglia of the EXtraordinarY Kids Clinic at the University of Colorado was kind enough to provide her expert recommendations for making the materials more accurate and more valuable for parents. Dr. Wylie Hembree of Columbia University helped me to revise the descriptions of puberty and of the various male hormone cycles into clear explanations for lay people of extraordinarily complex mechanisms. I was provided karyotype illustrations for the publication by the University of Wisconsin and by Susan Howell of the University of Colorado.

I must also thank some family members for lending me their expertise. My brother, Aaron, who has authored a number of local history books, encouraged me to develop a research, writing, publication, and "marketing" outline, which gave me the discipline and structure to carry out this year-long project. My sister, Patti, who has had a long career in publishing, provided editing and graphics support. She recommended Dorie McClelland, whose design work (and patience with my inexperience) has insured that this book is the professional product that I dreamed of producing.

My husband, Al, has provided the monetary and psychological support while I worked on my computer. He avoided commenting on the appearance of dust bunnies in the corner, and sometimes distracted, haphazard meals because I was too busy to shop. And John, who lives with Klinefelter syndrome and its challenges as he works on becoming an independent adult, provided my reason each day for wanting to complete this book.

The people that I must acknowledge most of all, however, are the 800+ respondents to the online survey that was posted internationally on a variety of SCA websites and list-serves. I did provide an earnest explanation of who I was and why I was asking for fairly personal information about their development and psychological functioning, or that of their loved ones. I was struck by how candid the replies were, whether they chose to remain anonymous or gave me their e-mail addresses. I realized through reading the open-ended responses that these persons were truly grateful that someone cared enough about this little-known and poorly understood group of disorders to go to the extraordinary effort of developing a published guide. The survey provided valuable information about what is most important to potential readers, and therefore provided a true focus for my writing. This book is dedicated to the individuals and families that participated and who told me so much about themselves and about the impact of SCA on their lives.

Resources

This listing of resources is not comprehensive, and provides only starting places for web-based research into organizations and list-serves that can assist with X and Y Chromosome Variation information, education and support services. Links were tested at operational at the time of publication.
KS&A stands for Knowledge, Support and Action. The group was founded as Klinefelter Syndrome and Associates, but now provides education and advocacy for all X and Y chromosome aneuploid conditions including XYY and XXX. Provides periodic family conferences, scientific meetings, an 800 number, and a website with numerous educational offerings including webinars. www.genetic.org
AAKSIS (American Association for Klinefelter Syndrome Information and Support) provides an 800 number for information and collaborates with KS&A on family conferences. www.AAKSIS.org

http://www.klinefeltersyndrome.org A website operated by Stefan Schwarz, who was diagnosed in early adulthood after a lifetime of learning disabilities and puzzling emotional problems. Provides support group information, links to e-mail lists and international support organizations and websites.
www.47xxy.com A website created and operated by a Canadian who was diagnosed in adulthood. Also provides information translated into French and Russian, as well as international resources.
Turner Center Danish Center for information on X and Y chromosomal anomalies. Provides information in English at: http://www.turnercenteret.dk/engelsk including texts of major academic journal articles. Information also available in Danish, French and German.
XXYY Project Information and advocacy, family conferences, and a website in English, German and French for families with boys and men who have 48,XXYY. http://xxyysyndrome.org/english.php

Triple-X Syndrome e-mail groups:
http://groups.yahoo.com/group/raregeneticdisorders
http://health.groups.yahoo.com/group/trisomyx
Tetrasomy and Pentasomy X e-mail group: http://www.tetrasomy.com
International Groups (This is not necessarily comprehensive. International resources are also available at www.klinefeltersyndrome.org and www.47xxy.org)

(Australia) http://klinefeltersyndrome.org/australia.htm
(Canada-French language) http://www3.sympatico.ca/ppicard1
(Germany) http://klinefelter.de/cms
(Japan) http://www.tokyo-med.ac.jp/genet/ks/indexj.html
(Netherlands) http://oud.klinefelter.ni
(Norway) http://klinefelter.no
(Spain) http://gamklinefelter.iespana.es/indes.htm
(U.K.) http://ksa-uk.co.uk
(U.K.) http://www.klinefelter.org.uk

EXtraordinarY Kids Clinic, University of Colorado, Aurora, CO. The only clinic of its kind, a university-based multi-specialty clinic offering comprehensive assessment and treatment by developmental pediatrics, endocrinology, psychology, speech pathology, genetics, other specialists. Medical insurance can be used to pay part of the cost of consultations. Appointment information: **(720)777-8361.** http://www.childrenscolorado.org/conditions/behavior/xychromosome.aspx

NORD (National Association for Rare Disorders) www.rarediseases.org
Genetic Alliance www.geneticalliance.org
Wrightslaw www.wrightslaw.com A leading resource for special education law and methods
GRASP (Global and Regional Asperger Syndrome Partnership) www.grasp.org
CHADD (Children and Adults with Attention Deficit/Hyperactivity Disorder) www.chadd.org
ILRU (Independent Living Centers Directory) The term 'center for independent living' means a consumer-controlled, community-based, private nonprofit agency that is designed and operated within a local community by individuals with disabilities and provides an array of independent living resources, including advocacy and referrals, vocational assistance, and legal services associated with benefits eligibility. The website provides links to centers in the U.S., Canada, and a number of other countries as well as other disability information and resources. www.ilru.org

Bibliography

Abramsky, L., and Chapple, J., "47,XXY (Klinefelter Syndrome) and 47,XYY: Estimated Rates of and Indication for Postnatal Diagnosis and Implications for Prenatal Counseling." *Prenatal Diagnosis* 17:No 4 (1994): 363–368.

Baker, S.R., Northeast, A.D.R., Berry, A.C., and Burnand, K.G., "Venous Ulceration in Males with Sex Chromosome Abnormalities." *Journal of the Royal Society of Medicine* 86 (January 1993): 24–25.

Bender, Bruce, A., Harmon, Robert J., Linden, Mary G., and Robinson, Arthur, "Psychosocial Adaptation of 39 Adolescents with Sex Chromosome Abnormalities." *Pediatrics* 96:No 2 (1995): 302–308.

__________, Linden, Mary G., and Robinson, Arthur, "Neuropsychological Impairment in 42 Adolescents with Sex Chromosome Abnormalities." *American Journal of Medical Genetics (Neuropsychiatric Genetics)* 48 (1993): 169–173.

Boada, Richard; Janusz, Jennifer; Hutaff-Lee, Christa; and Tartaglia, Nicole, "The Cognitive Phenotype in Klinefelter Syndrome: A Review of the Literature Including Genetic and Hormonal Factors." *Developmental Disabilities Research Reviews* 15 (2009): 284–294.

Bojesen, Anders; Juul, Svend; Birkebaek, Niels H., and Gravholt, Claus H., "Morbidity in Klinefelter Syndrome: A Danish Register Study Based on Hospital Discharge Diagnoses." *Journal of Clinical Endocrinology and Metabolism* 91:No 4 (2006);1254–1260.

__________, Kristensen, K., Birkebaek, N., Fedder, J., et al. "The Metabolic Syndrome is Frequent in Klinefelter's Syndrome and Is Associated with Abdominal Obesity and Hypogonadism." *Diabetes Care* 29:No 7 (July 2006):1591–1598.

Boone, K., Swerdloff, R., Miller, B.L., et al. "Neuropsychological profiles of adults with Klinefelter Syndrome." *Journal of the International Neuropsychological Society* 7 (2001): 446–456.

Bruining, H., Swaab, H., Kas, M., and van Engeland, H., "Psychiatric Characteristics of a Self-Selected Sample of Boys with Klinefelter Syndrome." *Pediatrics* (2009) http://www.pediatrics.org/cgi/content/full/123/5/e865

Forabosco, A., Percesepe, A., and Santucci, S., "Incidence of non-age-dependent chromosomal abnormalities: a population-based study on 88965 amniocenteses." *European Journal of Human Genetics* 17 (2009):897–903. http://www.nature.com/ejhg/journal/v17/n7/full/ejhg2008265a.html

Geschwind, Daniel H. and Dykens, Elisabeth, "Neurobehavioral and Psychological Issues in Klinefelter Syndrome." *Learning Disabilities Research and Practice* 19:No 3 (2004):166–173.

Giedd, J., Clasen, L., Wallace, G., Lenroot, R., et al. "XXY (Klinefelter Syndrome): A Pediatric Quantitative Brain Magnetic Resonance Imaging Case-Control Study." *Pediatrics* (2007) http://www.pediatrics.org/cgi/content/ful/119/1/e232

Gotz, M., Johnstone, E.C., and Ratcliffe, S.G., "Criminality and Antisocial Behavior in Unselected Men with Sex Chromosome Abnormalities 29 No 4 (1999):953–962.

Itti, E., Gaw Gonzalo, T., Pawlikowska-Haddal, K., Boone, K.B., et al. "The Structural Brain Correlates of Cognitive Deficits in Adults with Klinefelter Syndrome." *Journal of Clinical Endocrinology and Metabolism* (January 2006) doi:10.1210/jc.2005–1596.

Lee, N.R., Wallace, G., Clasen, L., Lenroot, R., et al. "Executive Function in Young Males with Klinefelter (XXY) Syndrome with and without Comorbid Attention-Deficit/Hyperactivity Disorder." *Journal of the International Neuropsychological Society* 17 (2011):1–9.

Leggett, V., Jacobs, P., Nation, K., et al. "Neurocognitive outcomes of individuals with a sex chromosome trisomy: XXX, XYY or XXY: a systematic review." *Developmental Medicine and Child Neurology* 52 (2010):119–129.

Lenroot, R., Lee, N.Raitano, and Giedd, J., "Effects of Sex Chromosome Aneuploidies on Brain Development: Evidence from Neuroimaging Studies." *Developmental Disabilities Research Reviews* 15 (2009):318–327.

Linden, M., Bender, B., and Robinson, A., "Intrauterine Diagnosis of Sex Chromosome Aneuploidy." *Obstetrics and Gynecology* 87:No 3 (March 1996):468–475.

__________, "Sex Chromosome Tetrasomy and Pentasomy." *Pediatrics* 96: No 4 (October, 1995):672–682

Mazzocco, Michele and Ross, Judith, eds., *Neurogenetic Developmental Disorders: Variation of Manifestation in Childhood.* (Cambridge: MIT Press, 2007), 48–72, 367–491.

Neilsen, J. and Pelsen, B., "Follow-up 20 years later of 34 Klinefelter males with karyotype 47,XXY and 16 hypogonadal males with karyotype 46,XY." *Human Genetics* 77 (1987):188–192.

Paduch, D., Fine, R., Bolyakov, A., and Kiper, J., "New Concepts in Klinefelter Syndrome." *Current Opinion in Urology* 18 (2008):621–627.

Patwardhan, A.J., Eliez, S., Bender, B., Linden, M., Reiss, A., "Brain Morphology in Klinefelter Syndrome: Extra X chromosome and testosterone supplementation." *Neurology* 54 No 12 (June 2000):1–10.

Rogol, Alan and Tartaglia, Nicole, "Considerations for Androgen Therapy in Children and Adolescents with Klinefelter Syndrome (47,XYY)." *Pediatric Endocrinology Reviews* 8 Supp. 1 (December 2010):145–150.

Ross, J., Zeger, M., Kushner, H., Zinn, A., et al. "An Extra X or Y Chromosome: Contrasting the Cognitive and Motor Phenotypes in Childhood in Boys with 47,XYY Syndrome or 47,XXY Klinefelter Syndrome." *Developmental Disabilities Research Reviews* 15 (2009):309–317.

Schiff, J., Palermo, G., Veeck, L., Goldstein, M., Rosenwaks, Z., and Schlegel, P., "Success of Testicular Sperm Extraction and Intracytoplasmic Sperm Injection in Men with Klinefelter Syndrome." *Journal of Clinical Endocrinology and Metabolism* 90 No 11 (2005):6263–6267.

Shear, N. and Lester, R., "Recurrent Leg Ulcerations as the Initial Clinical Manifestations of Klinefelter Syndrome." *Archives of Dermatology* 131 No 2 (February, 1995):230–232.

Stewart, D., Bailey, J., Netley, C., Rovet, J., and Park, E., "Growth and Development from Early to Midadolescence of Children with X and Y Chromosome Aneuploidy: The Toronto Study." *Birth Defects: Original Article Series,* 22 No 3 (1986):119–182.

Swerdlow, A.J., Higgins, C.D., Minouk, J., Shoemaker, J., Wright, Al, and Jacobs, P., "Mortality in Patients with Klinefelter Syndrome in Britain: A Cohort Study." *Journal of Clinical Endocrinology and Metabolism* 90(2005):6516–6522.

Tartaglia, N., Howell, S., Sutherland, A., Wilson, R., and Wilson, L., "A Review of Trisomy X (47,XXX)." *Orphanet Journal of Rare Diseases* 5 No 8 (2010): http://www.ojrd.com/content/5/1/8

__________, Cordeiro, L., Howell, S., Wilson, R., Janusz, J., "The Spectrum of the Behavioral Phenotype in Boys and Adolescents with 47,XXY (Klinefelter Syndrome)." *Pediatric Endocrinology Reviews* 8 Supp 1 (December 2010):151–159.

Visootsak, J., Rosner, B., Dykens, E., Tartaglia, N., and Graham, J., "Behavioral Phenotype of Sex Chromosome Aneuploidies: 48,XXYY, 48,XXXY, and 49,XXXXY." *American Journal of Medical Genetics Part A* (207):1198–1203.

Visootsak, J., and Graham, J.M., "Klinefelter Syndrome and other Sex Chromosomal Aneuploidies." *Orphanet Journal of Rare Diseases* 1 No 42 (2006): http://www.ojrd.com/content/1/142

Van Rijn, S., Swaab, H., and Aleman, A., "Social Behavior and Autism Traits in a Sex Chromosomal Disorder: Klinefelter Syndrome." *Journal of Autism and Developmental Disorders* (2008) http://www.springerlink.com/content/g68408vq74752421/

Warwick, M., Doody,G., Lawrie, S., et al. "Volumetric magnetic resonance imaging study of the brain in subjects with sex chromosome aneuploidies." *Journal of Neurology, Neurosurgery, and Psychiatry* 66 No 5 (May, 1999):628–632.

Wilson, Lennie, "Racial and ethnic distribution of identified males with XXY found through Fragile X Screening." Private communication. October 21, 2009.

Virginia Cover

In the 1980s at age 37, Virginia Isaacs Cover became pregnant with her second son. Amniocentesis revealed a prenatal diagnosis of Klinefelter Syndrome, or 47,XXY. Cover and her husband had the best genetic counseling available at the time in addition to access to copies of available research studies from the Stony Brook University's medical library through a highly qualified geneticist. Together with a pediatric endocrinologist, the geneticist painted a thorough picture of what might be a mildly disabling condition. Although there is now slightly more information available about the condition, much of it on the Internet, there is still a general lack of awareness among health care and education professionals as well as the general population. As the parent of a child with Klinefelter Syndrome, and with an advanced degree in social work, Ms. Cover has distilled two decades of experience and study into an authoritative guide for families and individuals affected by X and Y chromosome variations.

She draws on her years of experience as a parent, as an advocate, and as a social worker involved with children and adults with developmental disabilities, to research psychosocial and medical issues affecting this population. This guide provides a lifespan approach to the three trisomy conditions, Klinefelter Syndrome, Trisomy X, and 47,XYY Syndrome, as well as their less common Tetrasomy and Pentasomy variations. *Living with Klinefelter Syndrome (*47,XXY*) Trisomy X (*47,XXX*) and* 47,XYY provides clear explanations of the genetics involved in these conditions, diagnosis and disclosure, development from infancy through early adulthood, potential health issues, and educational and psychosocial considerations.

Ms. Cover grew up in Minnesota and earned an M.S.W. from the School of Social Work at the University of Michigan. Throughout her career, she has worked as a health care administrator and social worker, providing services to children and adults with special health care needs, and developing community-based programs for persons with chronic medical conditions including genetic disorders and developmental disabilities. She currently maintains a private practice focused on developing services for young adults with developmental disabilities. Ginnie coordinates support groups for persons with sex chromosome aneuploidy; serves as Director of Education for KS&A (Knowledge, Support and Action), a national advocacy and education organization; and provides educational presentations on X and Y chromosome variations to a broad range of audiences. She lives on Long Island in New York with her husband and their two Yorkshire Terriers.

Printed in Great Britain
by Amazon